A COMPLETE G⸻
DIAGNOSIS, ⸻

As many as 28 million Ameri⸻ hearing loss. You, or someone you love, may ⸻ them. This helpful, comprehensive, and compassionate sourcebook, written in plain English and filled with the real-life experiences of people of all ages, deals with what can be done medically to treat hearing loss, what tips and strategies can improve daily living, and what new devices and technologies are available. Now, the frustration, pain, and sense of loss associated with any degree of hearing problem can be greatly relieved. Here you'll find the latest information on:

* Medical treatments, from surgery to "invisible" hearing aids
* Strategies to make your home safe and comfortable, such as smoke detectors you can "hear" and "hearing ear" dogs
* How to prevent further hearing loss
* Devices to help you enjoy television, movies, and going out
* Coping with hearing loss on the job, in personal relationships, and with family and friends
* Plus comprehensive listings of suppliers, support groups, organizations, and catalogs

THE HEARING LOSS SOURCEBOOK

CAROL TURKINGTON is a freelance writer specializing in medical topics. A former editor at Duke University Medical Center, she is the author of numerous health books and has written for *Vogue, Self,* the *New York Times, Psychology Today, Good Housekeeping,* and many other publications. She lives in Lancaster, Pennsylvania.

By the Same Author

The Encyclopedia of Deafness and Hearing Disorders
Making the Prozac Decision: A Guide to Antidepressants
12 Steps to a Better Memory

THE
HEARING LOSS
SOURCEBOOK

A COMPLETE GUIDE TO COPING WITH HEARING LOSS AND WHERE TO GET HELP

Carol A. Turkington

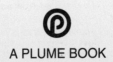

A PLUME BOOK

PUBLISHER'S NOTE
The ideas, procedures, and suggestions contained in this book are not intended as a substitute for consulting with your physician. All matters regarding your health require medical supervision.

PLUME
Published by the Penguin Group
Penguin Books USA Inc., 375 Hudson Street,
New York, New York 10014, U.S.A.
Penguin Books Ltd, 27 Wrights Lane,
London W8 5TZ, England
Penguin Books Australia Ltd, Ringwood,
Victoria, Australia
Penguin Books Canada Ltd, 10 Alcorn Avenue,
Toronto, Ontario, Canada M4V 3B2
Penguin Books (N.Z.) Ltd, 182–190 Wairau Road,
Auckland 10, New Zealand

Penguin Books Ltd, Registered Offices:
Harmondsworth, Middlesex, England

First published by Plume, an imprint of Dutton Signet, a division of Penguin Books USA Inc.

First Printing, May, 1997
10 9 8 7 6 5 4 3 2 1

 REGISTERED TRADEMARK—MARCA REGISTRADA

LIBRARY OF CONGRESS CATALOGING-IN-PUBLICATION DATA:
Turkington, Carol.
    The hearing loss sourcebook : a complete guide to coping with hearing loss and
where to get help / Carol A. Turkington.
        p.   cm.
    Includes index.
    ISBN 0-452-27577-6
    1. Deafness—Popular works. 2. Patient education.   I. Title.
RF291.35.T87   1997
617.8—dc21   96-37793
                                                                          CIP

Printed in the United States of America
Set in New Baskerville
Designed by Leonard Telesca

For Bert

Contents

Acknowledgments   ix
Introduction   xi

1. What Is Hearing Loss?   1
2. Diagnosing a Hearing Loss   13
3. Children and Hearing Loss   21
4. Hearing Loss in Adulthood   45
5. Noise and Hearing Loss   61
6. Do You Need a Hearing Aid?   71
7. Other Assistive Devices   107
8. How to Adapt to a Hearing Loss   136

Appendix: Organizations and Resources   145
Glossary   156
Index   163

Acknowledgments

The creation of any book always involves many people, and this one is no exception to that rule. While it's not possible to mention everyone who has worked with me on this book, I would like to thank staff members at Gallaudet University's library, public relations office, university press, and information center.

I also appreciate the efforts of countless folks from national organizations, services, and government agencies who work with deaf and hard-of-hearing individuals, including the Cochlear Implant Information Center, AT&T, National Captioning Institute, the FDA, Self Help for Hard of Hearing People, and Telecommunications for the Deaf, Inc.

Thanks also to staffers at the National Library of Medicine and the medical libraries of Hershey Medical Center, the University of Pennsylvania Medical Center and Reading Speech and Hearing Center, and the National Institutes of Health.

I'd also like to thank Deirdre Mullane at Dutton for her expert editorial guidance and Bert Holtje of James Peter Associates for his valuable support.

Introduction

One out of every ten Americans experiences some degree of hearing loss, and since a normal part of aging includes the gradual loss in hearing ability, hearing loss will only increase as our country's population ages. Already, ten million older Americans have been diagnosed with this type of age-related hearing loss.

Despite the prevalence of hearing loss, there are very few books available that offer detailed information in an accessible way. Whether you have trouble hearing or you are concerned about someone else who does, this book is for you. It's designed to provide the most up-to-date information about the symptoms, diagnosis, and treatment of hearing loss.

In each chapter, we'll explore strategies and tips for coping with hearing loss, illuminated by personal anecdotes from folks who've been there. You'll learn of the many causes of hearing loss, including viruses, bacteria, substance abuse, and medications. This book discusses a number of ear diseases that can cause hearing loss as well.

You'll also discover the real danger that excess environmental noise represents and how to protect yourself from ear damage. And you'll learn of laws designed to protect your hearing and what you can do to make your job a safer place.

Because so many Americans who need hearing aids aren't getting them—or don't wear them when they do—an important part of this book discusses the newest types of hearing aids and assistive devices now available on the market. Some of the newest versions have been designed to be almost invisible and are far more comfortable to wear. Many now do a much better job at screening out unwanted background noise.

For those interested in more information about any particular aspect of hearing loss, an extensive appendix in the back of the book includes a complete list of organizations and resources, including associations, research groups and schools. A glossary is also included to help readers understand often-used technical terms.

1

What Is Hearing Loss?

Jill Jones, 42, first recognized that she had a hearing problem as a college student, when she began to have trouble hearing on the phone. Now unable to hear without hearing aids, she believes her severe hearing loss may actually have begun in childhood. Like many people with hearing problems, she was never tested when she was a child. "I think it's the isolation that bothers me most," Jill feels. "If I'm talking with friends and I'm having trouble following the conversation, people get tired of repeating themselves. They start to exclude me. I know when they start to shut me out, and I can tell you it's a very lonely feeling."

It's estimated that as many as 28 million Americans of all ages have some form of hearing loss ranging from mild to severe. At some point almost all of us will develop a hearing problem if we live long enough. For most of us, age-related hearing loss begins between ages 55 and 65, although it can begin as soon as the early thirties in men and the late thirties in women. Age-related hearing loss, known as *presbycusis*, is not a symptom of any particular problem—it's simply a function of age. Of course, hearing loss can occur at any age—you can be born with unlucky genes, you can contract a childhood disease that affects your ears, or you can injure your hearing through an accident.

Symptoms of Hearing Loss

If a friend or family member is starting to have problems hearing, you may start to notice changes in the person's personality and attitude. A child in a classroom may begin to stop paying attention, and her grades may start to drop. An adult may begin to feel cut off. He may miss parts of conversations and begin to think people are talking about him, or become hostile and accuse others of mumbling.

It's not uncommon for people with failing hearing not to realize the gradual decline is taking place. Many people still fear that poor hearing is a sign of old age or that wearing a hearing aid carries a social stigma. Quite often they react with disbelief or hostility when the possibility of hearing loss is pointed out to them.

"I didn't want to believe that I wasn't able to hear as well as I used to," said David, a 45-year-old technician. "But then our young daughter would cry in her room, and my wife would get up to see what was wrong—but I hadn't heard a thing. Or our cat would cry at the door to come in, and I couldn't hear her. My wife would say, 'Don't you hear that?' and I'd have to admit that I didn't."

There are other, less obvious, signs of potential hearing loss that warrant a check-up by an ear specialist.

Speech deterioration

Since your ears help you modulate loudness and pronunciation, it's not surprising that a hearing loss can seriously affect the quality of human speech. If you begin to slur words or drop word endings (or if your speech sounds oddly "flat"), this could be a sign that you aren't hearing correctly.

Fatigue

Everyone gets tired now and then, but if you start to notice that you often feel exhausted or irritable while listening to a conversation or a speech, your fatigue might be caused by straining to hear what's being said.

Indifference

If you can't hear conversation, it's easy to feel depressed and disinterested. What many people with hearing loss discover is that although folks in a group will make an initial effort, all too often they eventually decide it's too much trouble to speak loudly and clearly. Unintentionally, people with a hearing problem might find themselves being excluded from group conversations.

"Most people don't adjust their voices to your hearing problem," says Bob, a 55-year-old manager. "Even if they know you have a hearing problem, it seems as if they just can't be bothered. Or maybe it's just that they don't know *how* to speak so I can hear."

Social withdrawal

Not being able to hear what's being said and sensing that others don't have the patience to try to communicate can make people decide it's all just too much trouble. Many people who are beginning to lose their hearing feel that it's easier to avoid social situations in order to avoid potential embarrassment.

Insecurity

Knowing that it's easy to make mistakes in communication when your hearing isn't as good as it might be leads some people to develop a real fear of making errors. No matter how well or how poorly we hear, no one likes to say or do things that might be held up to ridicule or that make us feel foolish. Not being able to follow the flow of conversation means that it's much easier to misinterpret what's being said and either to answer a wrong question or say something completely unrelated to the topic.

"My husband is very good at pretending," says Helen, 48. "He'll nod his head and seem as if he's following along perfectly. I know he hasn't heard a word, but as long as he doesn't really volunteer information, he figures he's not going to make a fool of himself. But what that really means is that he's missing out on a lot of good conversations."

The symptoms of a hearing loss vary quite a lot from one person to the next. However, there are some basic signs of significant ear damage that indicate it's time to go see an ear specialist. These symptoms have been compiled by the National Hearing Aid Society:

- Visible deformity of the ear present since birth or as the result of trauma
- Drainage from the ear within the previous three months
- Sudden or rapidly progressive hearing loss
- Acute or chronic tinnitus (ringing in the ear) or dizziness
- Visible ear wax build-up or a foreign object in the ear canal requiring immediate attention
- Pain or discomfort in the ear

How We Hear

What actually goes wrong with the ear when you can't hear? Because of the complexity of the hearing mechanism, the problem could be due to one of a host of reasons. Let's look at some details about the physical structure of your ear and how the whole hearing process works.

Your ear is divided into three main parts: the outer, middle, and inner ear. The outer ear includes the part of the ear you can see, called the *pinna*, which serves as a sort of funnel to direct sound into the ear canal. This canal extends about an inch into your head and is designed to protect the fragile eardrum. It's responsible for boosting the loudness of pitch important for understanding speech.

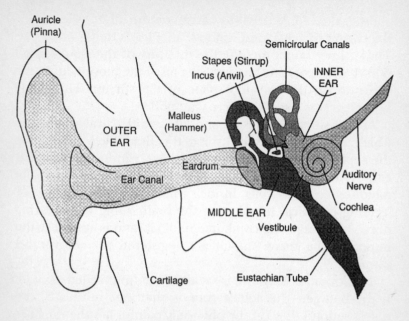

Diagram of the ear.

Hearing is a complex process that begins when sounds, which are actually vibrations, travel into the ear and along the ear canal to the eardrum, the entrance to the middle ear. The eardrum, or tympanum, is an important part of the hearing mechanism. Thin and pearly translucent, its inner layer is made up of mucous membrane covered by skin. Tiny blood vessels supply oxygen to the eardrum, which is normally almost transparent; when an infection is present, the vessels become inflamed and engorged, making the entire eardrum red and opaque.

When sound strikes the sensitive eardrum, it is passed along to three tiny bones, called ossicles, on the other side. The smallest bones in the human body are called the hammer (malleus), anvil (incus), and stirrup (stapes). (Interestingly, they are full size at birth.) The hammer is the first of the three bones, joined to the inside of the eardrum; next comes the anvil, joined to the hammer on one side and by another delicate joint to the stirrup on the other. The base of the stirrup fills the "oval window" that leads to the inner ear. These three bones amplify the intensity of the sound vibrations by compressing and focusing all of the movement in the eardrum on the tiny foot plate of the stirrup. The whole process acts as a sort of internal amplifier.

As the stirrup moves, it also vibrates the oval window to which it is attached, disturbing the fluid-filled channel of the cochlea on the other side of the oval window in the inner ear. As the cochlea moves, it stimulates the thousands of microscopic hair cells inside, which are responsible for sending electrical impulses to the brain along the "hearing nerve." Through this combination of vibrations and electrical impulses, the many stimuli are registered as recognizable sounds.

The loudness of sound is measured in units called decibels (dB). Between the softest sounds that can be heard and noises so loud they can be physically painful lies the range of sound you use for conversation.

Balance Mechanism

There are other structures in the inner ear that don't contribute to hearing but serve very important purposes. Located deep within the inner ear is a windy maze of passages called the labyrinth. The rear section is a series of three semicircular canals at right angles to each other, connected to a cavity called the vestibule. These canals contain hair cells that are constantly bathed in fluid, some of which are sensitive to gravity and acceleration, and others to the position and movement of the head. This information is registered by the cells and sent along nerve fibers to the brain. Problems within these tiny semicircular canals may cause dizziness, vertigo, and other balance problems. This is why so many problems in the hearing mechanism found in this area are accompanied by dizziness and vertigo.

Finally, the eustachian tube, a sort of "ventilation channel," runs forward and down into the back of the nose. Although the eustachian tube is normally closed, it opens when you yawn and swallow. The eustachian tube allows you to replace air absorbed by middle-ear tissues, drain off fluid, and equalize air pressure inside and outside the middle ear. (When your ears pop during a steep climb, this is really your eustachian tube opening.)

How Big a Problem Is Hearing Loss?

There are almost as many different types and gradations of hearing loss as there are people who can't hear. Hearing loss can be classified in three ways: by degree, configuration, and type. *Degree* and *configuration* refer to the range and volume of sounds that cannot be heard. *Type* refers to the part of the auditory system that has been affected.

Degree of Hearing Loss

The *degree* of hearing loss is the most common way to describe a person's hearing loss. There are four different levels: mild, moderate, severe, and profound.

If you have a *mild* hearing loss (15–30 decibel loss), you may lose track of the conversation or have problems hearing across a crowded room. You can't hear soft sounds, and you might have to ask people to repeat what they say. It's hard for you to hear in noisy situations.

A *moderate* hearing loss (35–55 dB) can make it difficult to hear others talk unless they speak loudly, and speech may not sound clear to you. You may find yourself asking people to repeat what they have said, and you might often misunderstand conversations.

If you have a *severe* hearing loss (60–90 dB), it can be very hard to understand speech, even in the quietest room. Many speech sounds are unclear, although vowels are easier to hear than consonants.

You won't be able to hear even very loud sounds (such as someone shouting) if you have a *profound* hearing loss (90 or above). Low pitches (such as vowels) might be the only sounds you can hear.

Although it's possible to have the same amount of hearing loss in both ears, most people hear better in one ear than the other. And most people with a hearing loss can hear *some* sounds even without a hearing aid.

The degree of hearing loss is strictly a medical and legal way to describe the variation in hearing from the norm. It does not deal with problems such as clarity of pitch perception, loudness, and so on, which also affect our hearing.

Configuration

The *configuration* of hearing loss is the range of pitch or frequency at which the loss occurs. Your hearing loss configuration influences how well you can hear speech. Normally, speech varies in loudness and pitch. Vowels have strong low-frequency sounds that can penetrate background noise fairly well, whereas consonants tend to be higher and weaker in pitch and fade out at a distance. Consonants are often obscured by background noise.

If you have a hearing loss, you probably hear some frequencies better than others, which can be a problem in understanding speech that involves a broad range of frequencies (especially higher ones). "I have a much harder time hearing the women in my family," explains George, a 52-year-old electrical engineer. "My son is no problem, but anyone with a high voice is impossible for me to make out."

Because of differences in the configuration of a hearing loss, two people with the same degree of hearing loss may hear an entirely different range of sounds, and configuration must also be considered in evaluating and treating a hearing loss.

Type of Hearing Loss

There are a number of ways to classify hearing loss, but many researchers agree on classifying the main kinds as conductive, sensorineural, mixed (a combination of conductive and sensorineural), or central. (In addition, a few people experience hearing loss as a result of a type of mental problem; this form of loss is known as *psychogenic* or *functional* hearing loss.)

Conductive hearing loss

Conductive hearing loss occurs when something is interfering with the transmission of sound to the inner ear. This problem can occur because of a simple blockage (such as ear wax or swelling from infection) or because of damage to the eardrum or the three bones of the middle ear. In an adult, this type of hearing loss also may be caused by the disease known as otosclerosis (*see Chapter 3*). A child with a conductive hearing loss has usually experienced several ear infections with a collection of sticky fluid in the middle ear.

Sometimes a conductive hearing loss is the result of damage to the eardrum or middle ear caused by sudden pressure changes (barotrauma) or by a punctured eardrum. Any blockage of the eustachian tube can also cause a conductive hearing loss. If you've ever had a severely stuffed nose and blocked ears during a cold, you know what this feels like. Most of the time a conductive hearing loss makes all sounds appear muffled.

Fortunately, there are all sorts of treatments for this type of problem, depending on the underlying reason. Surgery of the stapes (called a stapedectomy) may help people with some ear diseases. A hole in the eardrum or missing hearing bones can be corrected with reconstructive surgery as well.

Sensorineural hearing loss

Sensorineural hearing loss is a general term used to describe hearing problems from a number of conditions in which the sounds that reach the inner ear don't continue on to the brain because of problems with the structure of the inner ear. You may have heard this type of hearing problem referred to as "nerve deafness," but actually there isn't any damage to the acoustic (hearing) nerve itself. Sensorineural hearing loss is usually permanent and irreversible and tends to progress slowly. It can affect one or both ears.

Many people with a sensorineural hearing loss have difficulty understanding speech (known as *word discrimination*), even if the other person is speaking in a loud voice. (This is one reason why hearing aids may not help this type of problem.) In general, people with sensorineural hearing loss have trouble understanding speech because they can't hear certain frequencies of sound. If you have trouble hearing high-pitched sounds, you'll also have a hard time hearing the consonants *t*, *k*, and *s*, for example, because these sounds don't carry. You might also notice that you don't hear a sound at all at one level but that a slight increase in volume becomes painful. This is known as *recruitment.*

As we shall see in the next chapter, a wide variety of problems can lead to sensorineural hearing loss. In general, about five thousand infants every year experience this type of loss as a result of hereditary hearing problems, birth injury, or maternal infection. After birth, sensorineural hearing loss may be caused by damage to the delicate mechanisms of the inner ear after exposure to loud noise, which injures the sensory cells and nerve fibers. Other diseases causing this type of deafness include Meniere's disease, certain drugs, or viral infections. In fact, any disease that affects blood flow to the inner ear (such as diabetes, emphysema, heart problems, atherosclerosis, or kidney problems) can cause hearing loss.

Sensorineural loss caused by problems with the hearing centers of the brain may be caused by a stroke, head injury, or damage from a benign tumor on the hearing nerve (acoustic neuroma). As we get older, the most likely cause of a sensorineural hearing loss is related to changes in the ear due to the normal aging process. Known as presbycusis (*see Chapter 5*), this type of hearing loss is still not well understood by researchers. Unfortunately, there are some cases in which the cause for this sort of loss is simply not known.

Sensorineural hearing loss is far more difficult to treat than the conductive form, primarily because doctors just don't know enough about the ear structures involved. Hearing loss that is caused by a medical problem may be improved by treating the underlying condition. And as research into cochlear implants (*see Chapter 6*) progresses, there may be more that doctors can do.

Occasionally, some people have a *mixed hearing loss*, in which there is a combination of conductive and sensorineural loss that occurs in the outer or middle ear, as well as the inner ear.

Central hearing loss

A much rarer type of hearing problem is known as central hearing loss, caused not by problems with the ear structures themselves but with the signals as they travel through the ear passages or when they reach the brain itself. With this type of loss, it's not the sound level but the understanding of language itself that becomes difficult.

Scientists still don't know a great deal about central hearing loss. They do know that it may be caused by a high fever, exposure to loud noise, certain drugs, head injury, circulation problems, or tumors. There is no treatment for central deafness, although special auditory training helps some people.

Psychogenic hearing loss

Finally, functional (also called nonorganic or psychogenic) hearing loss refers to a loss caused primarily by psychological or emotional factors. Sometimes there is some slight damage in the ear, but the actual recorded hearing loss is usually much less than the patient reports.

This type of problem is often caused by anxiety resulting from emotional conflicts and is beyond the control of the patient. The person is not faking it but truly experiences a loss of hearing. In many cases a functional hearing loss can occur at the same time as a true organic hearing problem. This is called functional overlay. In order to treat this problem effectively, a hearing specialist must figure out the two different components of the hearing problem, using a patient history and hearing tests.

Another version of this type of hearing problem is the person with poor hearing on one side and normal hearing on the other. A person with this problem, called *unilateral functional deafness*, may claim not to hear even the loudest noises on the bad side in spite of good hearing on the opposite side. These inconsistencies help to establish a diagnosis.

A person with a psychogenic hearing loss is not able to hear during waking or sleep but is able to hear under hypnosis. This problem requires intervention first with a diagnosis by a hearing specialist and then with treatment by a mental health professional.

By now you may have decided that you or someone you care about may have some signs of hearing loss. The next step is to see a doctor and perhaps a hearing specialist to make sure there really is a hearing problem—and what may be the source of the problem. In the next chapter you'll learn what sort of specialists may be involved and what to expect during a hearing evaluation.

2

Diagnosing a Hearing Loss

Since there's no way for you to tell for sure if your hearing problem is related to presbycusis or one of the other causes, it's important to visit a doctor for a correct diagnosis as soon as you begin to have a problem. Of course, it's not really possible for you to accurately test your own hearing, but you can follow some guidelines to see if you have a problem. Take this simple test and see if you answer yes to any of these questions. Do you:

- Let your spouse or friend do most of your talking for you?
- Get tired after a long conversation?
- Notice friends seem to be avoiding conversations with you?
- Have to ask people to repeat what they say again and again?
- Often misunderstand others?
- Tune out when more than one person is talking?
- Nod your head as if you are following the conversation when you actually don't understand what has been said?

- Notice people seem embarrassed by your answers, as if they don't fit the questions?
- Have a ringing or roaring in your ears?
- Feel as if people are mumbling?

Here's an even simpler test of hearing loss: rub your thumb and forefinger together, about six to eight inches from your ear. If you can't hear the scratching noise, you may have a hearing problem.

It's especially important to see your doctor right away if you experience dizziness, ringing or roaring noises in your ears, pain, a feeling of pressure, or drainage, since these symptoms could be signs of a serious medical problem.

If you do suspect a hearing loss, you can either visit your family doctor first for a referral to a specialist or make an appointment yourself with an ear, nose, and throat specialist (ENT physician); other terms for these experts include *otolaryngologist* or *otorhinolaryngologist.* Some of these specialists limit their practice to the ears; they are known are *otologists.*

In fact, this initial physician visit is so important, the Food and Drug Administration requires that a licensed physician evaluate your hearing within six months of buying a hearing aid (unless you sign a waiver). If you go directly to a hearing aid dealer for an aid without first visiting your doctor, the dealer is legally obligated to advise you that it's not a good idea to sidestep the medical exam. This is because only a doctor can assess the possible *cause* of your hearing loss, which could be the sign of a significant medical problem or nothing more than an accumulation of wax that can be removed in the doctor's office.

The Doctor Visit

During your first medical visit, a doctor will take a detailed medical history of your hearing problems and look inside your ears with an otoscope, a lighted device used to examine the ear. He will be looking for any evidence of infection, blockage, or other problem in the ear canal or eardrum that might be causing your hearing problem. Next, you may be tested for balance and coordination problems in order to rule out any neurological ailments underlying your hearing loss. Your doctor also may use a tuning fork to see if it's possible to make a rough estimate about your ability to hear.

Don't expect your doctor to conduct the precise tests necessary to fit you with a hearing aid. This is usually performed by an audiologist—a professional trained in evaluating hearing. An audiologist is not a medical doctor but may have a doctorate in audiology and thus be referred to as "Dr." While an ENT specialist is highly trained in the pathology of the ear and fully understands medical and surgical techniques, most aren't trained in the special skills of hearing rehabilitation. Your ENT specialist may have an audiologist on staff, or you may be given a referral and asked to return once the testing is done. In any case, look for the initials CCC-A (Clinical Certificate of Competence—Audiology) in the audiologist's title, which indicates certification from the American Speech Language Hearing Association.

What the Audiologist Does

If your doctor detects signs of hearing loss, an audiologist will want to give you a complete examination and conduct a series of hearing tests. An audiologist is a licensed and/or certified professional trained to identify and measure hearing loss, and to rehabilitate those with hearing or speech problems. Audiologists are trained to determine where hearing loss occurs, and they can assess the effect of the loss on your ability to communicate.

An audiologist can recommend hearing aids and provide counseling and therapy to help you deal with hearing loss. He also offers hearing aid evaluation and orientation, auditory and speechreading training, and speech conservation.

Audiologists are not physicians and thus cannot treat infections or other ear diseases.

You'll find audiologists working in a wide variety of settings, including universities, hospitals, schools, medical offices, and private practices. When employed by a university, audiologists may teach, supervise clinical practice, and direct clinical services. At medical centers, hospitals, and rehabilitation agencies, they test hearing, including a pre- and postoperative evaluation of surgical patients. Community hearing and speech centers employ audiologists to work with adults and children as rehabilitation specialists to test hearing, select hearing aids, and help improve speech and reading skills. Referrals come from a wide variety of professionals, including otolaryngologists, neurologists, neurosurgeons, pediatricians, geriatricians, family doctors, and internists. In hospitals with acute-care pediatric nurseries, audiologists direct hearing screening programs for infants at risk for hearing problems. In addition, hospital audiologists often dispense hearing aids.

Since most school districts require some type of hearing screening for students, audiologists may serve as directors of these programs and work with teachers to help with special educational needs of students with hearing problems. In schools with special classes for those with hearing problems, audiologists equip and maintain classroom amplification systems. You may also find an audiologist working in a private practice with your physician (especially an otolaryngologist), where they will test hearing, evaluate ear function, and dispense hearing aids.

Recently, audiologists have begun branching out into private practice themselves, primarily to dispense hearing aids directly to clients with hearing problems. What distinguishes them from commercial hearing aid dealers is the in-depth professional rehabilitation programs they can offer their customers.

When you go for your visit with an audiologist, you'll find that she may use a variety of tests to determine your ability to hear and understand. Although these tests usually measure hearing abilities, an audiologist may also test your skill at interpreting gestures and facial expressions.

An audiologist routinely tests three aspects of your hearing: the *degree* of hearing ability, the *kind* of hearing loss, and the ability to *understand speech* under different conditions. He will usually provide these services:

- Hearing screening to see if you have a hearing loss
- Hearing evaluation through a set of tests to gauge the amount and degree of hearing loss
- Hearing aid evaluation to decide if a hearing aid is recommended and what type of device is the best choice for you
- Counseling to help you learn to communicate more effectively, and to cope with the practical and emotional aspects of living with a hearing loss

When you arrive for your appointment with an audiologist, you'll first be asked to give a detailed case history. After checking your ears with an otoscope to rule out infection or obstruction, you'll be given a pair of headphones. The hearing tests take place in a soundproof booth designed to screen out background noise.

First, the audiologist will administer a basic screening test called a pure-tone air-conduction test. The test evaluates how softly you can hear across the spectrum of frequencies and measures the lowest hearing level at which you can respond correctly to pure tones 50 percent of the time. During the test a series of tones (like musical notes) will be played through your headphones in one ear at a time. You'll be asked to respond by raising your hand or pushing a button each time you first hear the tone. You should raise your hand whenever you detect this tone, even if it is very faint, since the purpose of the test is to find the softest sound you can hear in all frequency ranges. Since hearing loss may occur at some frequencies but not others, it's important to determine how well you hear across all frequencies.

Pure tones are usually in octave or half-octave steps and cover the frequencies between 250 and 8,000 hertz (Hz). Because speech falls within this range, it is possible (in a limited way) to measure your ability to hear a conversation by testing with pure tones. The disadvantage of pure tones is that the sounds heard every day are not pure but complex.

When there is a large difference between your hearing ability in the two ears, the audiologist will mask the better ear to prevent it from responding and giving a false reading while the poorer ear is tested. The better ear is masked by presenting a band of noise through the earphone at about the same frequency as the one being tested.

Pure bone conduction

Next, the audiologist might remove the headphones for a pure bone-conduction test. Bone conduction is the process by which sounds are transmitted through the skull directly to the cochlea. This test assesses the sensitivity of the inner ear. For this test the audiologist will place a small vibrator behind your ear, or on your forehead, and again you will be asked to indicate which sounds you can hear.

The "air-bone gap" is the difference between how well you hear by air conduction and bone conduction. If you have normal bone-conduction results but significant hearing loss as measured by air-conduction tests, this indicates that your hearing loss is a conductive loss, not sensorineural. Therefore, you may be a candidate for surgical or medical treatment of your hearing loss.

Speech-reception (or speech-recognition) threshold test

Although pure tones may reveal the nature and extent of your hearing loss, they don't reveal the extent of communication problems. In addition to pure tone tests, a hearing evaluation often includes some measure of how sensitive you are to speech (or the lowest level at which speech can be heard). For this test the headphones are placed on your ears, and the audiologist reads (or plays a tape) of two-syllable words. As you repeat what you hear, the words gradually become fainter until the point when you can no longer hear the words. This is your speech-reception threshold.

Speech-discrimination (word-recognition) test

This test measures your ability to understand speech when it's loud enough for you to hear. In this test the audiologist is trying to find out how clearly you can discriminate one-syllable words while listening at a comfortable level. The test determines how well you can understand important sounds (primarily consonants) and measures how well you can discriminate speech at intensities 30 to 40 dB above your speech-reception threshold. You'll be read a list of about 50 one-syllable words and asked to repeat them.

Discrimination Score

Discrimination Score	Interpretation
90–100%	Excellent understanding of speech
80–89	Good understanding of speech
70–79	Fair understanding of speech
60–69	Poor understanding of speech
0–59	Markedly reduced understanding of speech

Acoustic-immitance tests

Most hearing tests can uncover the type and degree of hearing loss, but they may not diagnose specific ear diseases. Acoustic-immitance tests may be used in addition to hearing tests, since it's possible to have significant ear disease with little hearing loss. Unlike most hearing tests, acoustic-immitance tests can reveal middle-ear disorders without requiring active participation on the part of the client, and are therefore good for use with young children.

Immitance tests evaluate the middle ear, measuring the response of the eardrum, ossicles, and small muscles attached to the ossicles. The most common acoustic-immitance test is the tympanogram, a measure of eardrum stiffness as a function of air-pressure change. It can determine with fairly good accuracy whether there is fluid behind the eardrum, or if air pressure in the middle ear is abnormal. Another acoustic-immitance test is the acoustic-reflex test, which measures the reflex contraction of muscle in the middle ear.

What happens next

After your hearing tests have been completed, the audiologist will discuss whether or not a hearing aid would help. If these tests show you have a hearing problem in the middle or outer ear, your doctor might be able to correct the problem with medical treatment or surgery. However, if the loss is a result of problems in the inner ear (such as hearing loss that occurs with age), your only option may be a hearing aid. While an aid cannot restore normal function to your ears, it can significantly improve your hearing.

If the audiologist believes a hearing aid may be of help, you'll be asked to undergo a hearing aid evaluation. Further tests will help pinpoint which type of hearing aid is best for your particular type of hearing loss.

Your audiologist will write a report of the results of your test and forward them to your ENT specialist. You may request a copy of this report for your own records.

If your doctor finds that you do in fact have a hearing loss, you'll want to know what caused the problem. In the next chapters we'll discuss the different problems that can lead to hearing loss.

3

Children and Hearing Loss

*"I was born deaf because of some medication my mother took
when she was pregnant. It was especially hard on her because
she happened to be deaf, too. I guess they just didn't know the
risks back then."*

Albert, 66

The complexity of the ear means that it is vulnerable to
damage from a wide variety of sources—disease, genetic disorders, infection, noise, or accidents. Each age has its unique
susceptibility: the fetus, because the ear mechanism is under-
going rapid development; the child, vulnerable to a host of
ototoxic diseases; the adult, prey to the disintegration of the
ear due to normal aging.

Prenatal Causes of Hearing Loss

Loss of hearing from prenatal causes occurs in between 7 and
20 percent of deaf and hard-of-hearing people. Significantly,

most of these prenatal causes are preventable. The three major threats to the hearing mechanism of a woman's unborn baby are viral diseases, ototoxic drugs (drugs that can harm hearing), and a woman's health during pregnancy. Of these the biggest threat to prenatal ear development is viral disease contracted by a pregnant mother.

The most dangerous of all the viral diseases from the standpoint of hearing is rubella, though damage also can be caused by the mother's infection with influenza, mumps, toxoplasmosis (protozoan infection), cytomegalovirus (CMV), and herpes. In fact, almost any severe infection can damage the developing fetal hearing mechanism, especially during the first trimester, when the fetus seems to be especially vulnerable. Only the common cold appears to carry no threat to an unborn child's ears.

German Measles (Rubella)

A mother who contracts German measles during the first three months of pregnancy may give birth to a child with some degree of hearing loss. Typically, the pregnant woman experiences just a mild rash and fever, but she may have no symptoms at all and not even realize she has been infected. About one third of children born to mothers who contract rubella may be deaf, especially if it occurs in the first few months of pregnancy. However, there have been cases in which a baby sustained hearing loss when the mother contracted rubella as late as the seventh month of pregnancy.

The mother can also infect her baby long after she contracts rubella, since the virus may linger in her body and go on to injure an embryo that is conceived weeks or months after the infection appears to have subsided. In some cases, the child's deafness may be progressive, because the virus persists in the child's body after birth. Moreover, children who carry the virus for long periods after birth tend to suffer more severely than those from whom the virus disappears after birth.

Children affected by this type of deafness experience severe but incomplete injury to the organ of Corti, but they are seldom totally deaf. Their hearing problems are likely to be more noticeable in the higher frequencies.

The rubella virus was finally isolated in the mid-1960s, and by 1968 a successful vaccine was developed. Because this vaccine is widely available, rubella-related deafness is preventable. In fact, following the German measles epidemic of the 1960s, many states began to require women to be tested for rubella antibodies when applying for a marriage license.

Toxoplasmosis

Prenatal infection by toxoplasmosis can also lead to a hearing loss. Up to 45 percent of American women of reproductive age carry this organism, usually passed on by infected cats and their waste, and one baby out of every 800 will develop toxoplasmosis in the womb from an infected mother.

Infected pregnant women may experience fatigue and muscle pain, although there may be no symptoms at all. Your doctor can't confirm the disease unless you had a negative toxoplasmosis test early in your pregnancy and subsequently test positive for the infection. Although the disease can be treated with medication, early infection can lead to miscarriage. Fortunately, if you do become infected while pregnant, most likely your baby won't develop the infection, and of those babies who do, only 17 percent will experience a hearing loss. Most babies born with toxoplasmosis don't show evidence of the infection immediately, but many physicians advise drug treatment anyway.

Cytomegalovirus

Up to half of all children infected with CMV in the womb will have a bilateral, sensorineural hearing loss of varying severity. Discovered in 1956, cytomegalovirus (CMV) is a member of the herpes virus family; it's the largest, most complex virus known to infect humans. The virus doesn't usually cause any symptoms in healthy people, but it may set off symptoms like the common cold in a pregnant woman. Hearing loss in infants is most often profound, although some babies sustain milder losses.

Cytomegalovirus infection in the womb is now considered a possible cause of many previously unknown cases of nongenetic hearing loss. In fact, some studies suggest that CMV has replaced rubella as the most common viral cause of prenatal deafness. This could be because CMV is extremely common; about 80 percent of adults have antibodies to this virus in their blood, indicating a previous infection. CMV is acquired by close personal contact with bodily secretions of someone infected with CMV and is harmless to anyone but a developing fetus or those with weakened immune systems (such as AIDS patients).

Babies can become infected in the womb, during birth, or in the first few weeks of life. Women with toddlers who attend day care, where CMV is prevalent, are often infected. While young children rarely have symptoms, they excrete the virus in their urine and saliva for months to years. Anyone working in a child-care setting or with many diapered infants is likely to be exposed to CMV. It may also be transmitted from blood transfusions, since so many people (including blood donors) have CMV without symptoms (though many blood facilities now screen for the virus). Although most people are infected before adulthood, very few experience any signs of illness.

Almost all babies infected before birth are nonetheless born perfectly normal. Only about 10 percent of those infected in the womb become sick; of these 20 to 30 percent may die, and the rest will have permanent damage to various organs, including the brain, eyes, lungs, and liver. Many infants will have hearing problems. In addition, recent studies suggest that a small number of seemingly normal CMV-infected babies may develop problems later in life.

There is no cure for congenital CMV, because once the virus damages the baby before birth, antiviral drugs can't repair this damage. If you are pregnant and have other children in day care, experts suggest you should wash your hands well after changing diapers and wiping noses. Disposable wipes may be a good idea. If you are pregnant and concerned, you can request a test for CMV antibodies when you begin prenatal care. Babies born to mothers who have already contracted CMV are at less risk of congenital CMV infection.

Other Infections

Several other viruses, including herpes, mumps, and the flu, are all capable of damaging a newborn's hearing. Because the herpes simplex virus has been linked to hearing problems in infants born to women with an active lesion in the genital area during labor, many physicians perform a Caesarian section for women with active lesions at time of birth. A pregnant woman who contracts the flu or mumps during the first three months of pregnancy is at increased risk of giving birth to a child with a hearing loss.

Viruses aren't the only risk to unborn babies. If you contract a bacterial infection before giving birth, you can transmit the infection via the bloodstream to your baby, causing pneumonia or meningitis. Other infectious agents that might be in the amniotic fluid can be swallowed by the baby and then pumped up the eustachian tube into the middle ear to cause an ear infection.

By 1964 doctors recognized *group B Streptococcus* as a threat to a newborn's health and hearing. Today it is responsible for most of the serious illness in babies younger than two months old. Although there are several different groups of streptococci, group B seems to infect pregnant women and newborns. Group B strep occurs in soil and vegetation, and is found normally in humans and many animals. But between 4 to 40 percent of pregnant women (depending on the region of the country) seem to concentrate group B in the genital area. About half of these women will give birth to babies affected by group B strep. While almost all babies (99 percent) born to mothers with group B strep present in the vaginal area will be healthy, about one in 100 will have symptoms that can include a long-term hearing loss.

Most experts recommend screening all pregnant women for group B strep at 26 to 34 weeks of pregnancy. Some suggest giving antibiotics to all mothers with a positive group B strep culture during labor and delivery.

Syphilis

Syphilis, a venereal disease, can be transmitted from mother to child during pregnancy; it may cause an inner-ear hearing loss in the child either during the first two years of life or when the child reaches puberty. Thirty-five percent of babies affected by the disease will eventually go on to experience some degree of hearing loss. This eventual loss is hard to quantify, since the deafness may show up suddenly later in childhood (or even in adulthood). Children tend to experience sudden hearing loss in both ears; if it appears before age ten, the deafness is usually profound.

Syphilitic labyrinthitis is usually caused by congenital syphilis and results in a sudden, flat sensorineural hearing loss or a sudden increasing fluctuation of sensorineural hearing loss. Fortunately, incidences of congenital syphilis are today very rare. When they do occur, they can be treated with antibiotics.

Rh Factor Incompatibility

If you have Rh-negative blood and you give birth to a child with Rh-positive blood, you develop antibodies to Rh-positive blood in response. Though this will not harm your first baby, subsequent pregnancies carry a risk of damage to the baby's hearing mechanism when your antibodies attack the red blood cells of an Rh-positive child.

The incompatibility can injure the ears or nervous system of your newborn during the first few days of life, either directly or as a result of jaundice caused by the abnormal destruction of red blood cells at or shortly after birth. As hemoglobin is broken down, it produces bilirubin, which can cause jaundice as it accumulates in certain areas in the brain. The auditory system is one of the systems that is likely to be injured by this bilirubin build-up.

Massive transfusions for your baby, if done promptly, can ease the problem. Transfusions that are too little or too late may not prevent permanent injury to your baby's hearing mechanisms. Fortunately, hearing problems for newborns due to Rh-sensitization are becoming rare since the development of Rh (D) immune globulin. When injected into the mother 72 hours before delivery, the shot prevents 99 percent of the incidences of sensitization.

Cerebral Palsy

Cerebral palsy is a general term for nonprogressive disorders of movement, posture, or speech caused by brain damage during pregnancy, birth, or early childhood. Between two and six infants out of every 1,000 develop CP (mostly shortly before or after birth). Of these, between 25 and 30 percent will have hearing problems.

Cerebral palsy can result from a mother's infection that has passed to her unborn baby, from birth trauma, or from too much bilirubin in the baby's blood after birth. In the newborn, cerebral palsy can be caused by a head injury, encephalitis, or meningitis.

Loss of Oxygen

During birth, anoxia (loss of oxygen) and hypoxia (reduced oxygen) are the two most frequent causes of damage to the hearing *organ of Corti*. Any disturbance of the infant's breathing or circulation can interfere with the level of oxygen in the blood and brain, and a complete loss of oxygen within a body tissue can kill cells unless corrected quickly. Loss of oxygen can be caused by a long labor, heavy sedation of the mother, obstruction of the baby's respiratory passages with mucus, poor lung development, or congenital circulatory or heart defects. The only treatment is prevention of these conditions.

Ototoxic Drugs

Certain medications that affect the hearing mechanism are known as ototoxic drugs. If taken by a pregnant woman, these drugs may harm the hearing mechanism of the developing fetus. They are particularly damaging to the unborn child if taken during the sixth or seventh week of pregnancy.

- *Streptomycin* When the antibiotic streptomycin is given to a pregnant woman at any time, it can cause a sensorineural hearing loss in her baby ranging from a mild problem hearing high-frequency sounds to a severe hearing loss in both ears.
- *Alcohol* Fetal alcohol syndrome is a combination of birth defects caused when a pregnant woman drinks too much alcohol. It has been reported that fetal alcohol syndrome may cause a sensorineural or conductive hearing loss in up to 64 percent of infants born to alcoholic mothers. Although even small amounts of alcohol can harm a developing fetus, the syndrome appears when the mother consistently drinks at least two mixed drinks or two to three bottles of beer or glasses of wine daily during her pregnancy.
- *Aminoglycosides* The incidence of prenatal deafness resulting from this class of drugs (kanamycin, neomycin, gentamicin, tobramycin, and amikacin) is very low for most people. These drugs have been reported to cause hearing loss in infants only when mothers who took them had kidney problems and received diuretics (ethacrynic acid and furosemide) in addition to an aminoglycoside. It has been suggested that there may be a genetic susceptibility to hearing problems associated with this class of drugs.

CAN YOUR CHILD HEAR?

Your doctor may be highly trained to detect disease, but as parents you are around your children all the time and often simply sense when something doesn't seem right. If you suspect your child has a hearing loss, you could be right. Here are some guidelines.

At birth to three months, your baby should:

- *Look startled if there is a sudden loud noise*
- *Stir in sleep, wake up, or cry if someone makes a noise*
- *Recognize the sound of your voice, usually quieting down and becoming calm when your voice is heard*

At three to six months, your baby should:

- *Respond to your voice*
- *Move its eyes to search for an interesting sound*
- *Turn its eyes toward you when you call the child's name*

At six to twelve months, your baby should:

- *Turn toward you when you call his name from behind*
- *Turn toward an interesting sound*
- *Understand simple words like* no *and* bye-bye

If your baby doesn't respond in this way, contact your pediatrician. *The earlier your baby's hearing loss is diagnosed, the better for the child.* Insist on a hearing test if you have concerns. Don't hesitate to take your child to a hearing specialist if you aren't satisfied with your pediatrician's response to your questions.

Childhood Causes of Acquired Deafness

In addition to prenatal causes of deafness, many viral diseases during childhood also may affect the inner ear. Often in these cases only one ear is damaged, although it is possible for both ears to be affected.

Bacterial Infections

The inner ear may harbor infections that can lead to a severe or total loss of hearing. The infection usually reaches the inner ear via the connection between the inner ear and the cranial cavity. Once the infection reaches the inner ear, it may destroy the auditory nerve, the organ of Corti, and other parts of the delicate auditory structures.

Although far rarer, it's possible for typhoid fever or diphtheria toxins to affect the ear. These toxins can destroy the organ of Corti and its associated structures. Formerly a common cause of acquired deafness in the United States, massive immunizations against these diseases in this country have made these toxin-related deafness cases quite rare.

Ear infection (otitis media)

If you have young children, chances are you already know a great deal about ear infections, since these pesky problems are responsible for 30 million pediatrician visits each year in the United States. Almost all American children have at least one infection by the time they are six years old. Children are most likely to be affected before age two, since in early life the eustachian tube is shorter, straighter, narrower, and more horizontal, making it easier for bacteria to enter from the back of the throat. Some children have recurrent attacks through age 10. Many types of viruses and bacteria may lead to ear infections.

Infections of the middle ear (otitis media) occur in the cavity between the eardrum and the inner ear; they can produce pus, fluid, and hearing loss. A cold can cause swelling and blocking of the eustachian tube, the passage that connects the back of the nose to the middle ear. This tube may become blocked by the infection or by enlarged adenoids (lymphoid tissue between the back of the mouth and the esophagus, often associated with infections of the nose and throat). Fluid produced by the inflammation can't drain off through the eustachian tube and instead collects in the middle ear. This fluid accumulation allows bacteria and viruses drawn in from the back of the throat to breed, causing infection. Hearing loss may occur, but it usually disappears with treatment.

Acute ear infection causes a sudden, severe earache, deafness, tinnitus (ringing in the ear), sense of fullness, and fever. It can be harder to detect an ear infection in an infant, but you can suspect such a problem if the baby has a low-grade fever, a cold with thickened discharge, and a poor appetite, or if the baby is irritable, pulls her ears, shakes her head, and cries in the middle of the night. There may or may not be fluid draining from the ear.

Although acute ear infections are a fact of life during childhood, chronic infections are more serious, since they can cause permanent damage due to constant irritation. Unfortunately, a chronic condition may not cause enough discomfort to bring immediate diagnosis and treatment, but left uncorrected, chronic infection can cause permanent hearing damage.

A doctor diagnoses an ear infection by examining the ear with an otoscope. A sample of discharge may be taken to identify the organism responsible for the infection, although usually a doctor won't try to determine which bacteria are causing the infection since the tests require draining the middle ear and culturing the liquid. (These tests may be done on a hospitalized or very sick child.)

Until you can see your doctor, you can relieve some of the child's pain with nonprescription pain relievers or by placing a warm cloth or heating pad over the affected ear.

Before the development of antibiotics, these infections

were the single greatest cause of hearing loss. Today your doctor can treat acute infections with antibiotics (usually amoxicillin), although since the mid-1980s some strains of bacteria have acquired resistance to amoxicillin. If your child has both an ear infection and conjunctivitis, the cause is almost always *H. flu*, and the drug cefixime may be the better antibiotic choice.

Your doctor may also remove pus and skin debris from the affected ear, and prescribe antibiotic drops, if necessary. Ephedrine nose drops can help establish drainage of the ear in children. As long as the eardrum is unbroken, ear drops will not help because they cannot reach the affected area. Your physician may cut into the eardrum (a process called *myringotomy*) to relieve pressure during an ear infection. Once the infection has cleared, the eardrum will heal.

Chronic conditions are usually treated with antihistamines and decongestants if they are associated with nasal congestion or allergies. If the situation does not improve and the adenoids are affected, your doctor may recommend their removal.

RISKS FOR EAR INFECTIONS

A number of factors increase a child's likelihood of getting ear infections. Your child is at greater risk for each infection if he is:
- Younger than two years
- Bottle-fed
- Male
- Native American or Hispanic
- Living in crowded conditions
- Attending day care
- Suffers from allergies
- Exposed to household cigarette smoke

Meningitis

Hearing loss is a common complication of meningitis, a disease involving inflammation and infection of the outer covering of the brain (meninges). About 6 percent of children with bacterial meningitis experience a sudden, profound sensorineural deafness in both ears; some researchers have reported a higher rate of occurrence. Most cases occur in children under age five. This type of deafness is incurable. A prescription antibiotic called rifampin can prevent cases of Hib and meningococcal meningitis after exposure.

If your child has had bacterial meningitis, experts recommend that you take the child for a hearing test after recovery and for periodic retests for the following 12 months.

In the early 1900s bacterial meningitis was the most common clearly identified cause of acquired total deafness in children. Since then preventive shots (the Hib vaccine) have sharply reduced the incidence of the disease, and antibiotics have saved the lives of many children who have become infected. However, it's possible that a child may survive but still experience total destruction of the inner ear.

Scarlet fever

Also known as scarlatina, this acute infectious disease is caused by the streptococcus bacterium. It can lead to complications such as sinus infections that may be followed by ear abscesses and mastoiditis.

Spread by droplets in the air, scarlet fever gets its name from the reddish flush and rash it causes, in addition to a sore throat and high fever. Once a dangerous and common childhood disease, it is today fairly rare in the United States. It is believed that the reduced threat of the disease is due to a mysterious change in the virulence of the bacteria, not the development of drugs used to treat the condition. If this disease does infect a child, it is usually easily treatable if medication is started promptly.

Viral Infections

Viruses are common causes of sudden, high-frequency hearing problems in children. Because viruses are so small (much smaller than bacteria), they are carried to the ear directly from the bloodstream. They are capable of destroying the delicate hearing structures (such as the organ of Corti). The resulting hearing loss can be quite severe, but it does not usually worsen over time. There are a number of common viruses to watch for.

Chickenpox

This common, mild childhood infectious disorder has been known to cause sudden severe deafness in one ear. Chickenpox is caused by the varicella-zoster virus, a relative of the herpes family of viruses. After infection the virus lies dormant within nerve tissues and may erupt as herpes zoster (shingles) later in life. One episode of the viral disease confers lifelong immunity.

Chickenpox is heralded by a rash on the body, face, upper arms and legs, under the arms, inside the mouth, and sometimes in the bronchial tubes. Although children usually have only a slight fever, adults may become quite ill, with severe pneumonia and breathing problems. Complications include encephalitis (brain inflammation), which can lead to central hearing loss. While the incidence of deafness and other complications related to chickenpox is small, the American Academy of Pediatrics recommends that all children receive the recently approved vaccine against chickenpox.

Measles

This viral illness causes a rash and fever, and may lead to hearing problems or deafness as a result of complications of ear infections or encephalitis (brain inflammation). Though measles usually affects children, an attack may occur at any age.

Measles is spread by airborne droplets with an incubation

period of up to 11 days before symptoms appear. The illness can be transmitted during this period and up to one week after symptoms occur. Once very common around the world, today measles appears much less often in developed countries because of the availability of vaccinations against the disease.

Encephalitis

This term refers to an inflammation of the brain, which can lead to central hearing problems. The hearing loss is usually the result of problems within the brain, not with the hearing apparatus within the ear itself. Encephalitis is usually caused by an infection. Viruses are the most common, although the disease can result from many different kinds of chemicals or organisms. Two types of viruses can cause encephalitis: those (such as rabies) that invade the body but don't cause trouble until they reach the brain cells, and those (such as herpes simplex, herpes zoster, and yellow fever) that first harm non-nervous tissue and *then* invade brain cells.

Mumps

This acute viral disease is the most common cause of severe, one-sided deafness, which usually appears suddenly and may go unnoticed for days (or years) after it occurs since there is no pain or discomfort. Often a patient will say he only recently noticed deafness in one ear, but further investigation reveals that the deafness has in fact been present since an attack of mumps in childhood.

Deafness may occur when the mumps virus spreads to the lining of the brain and usually causes complete loss of hearing in one ear by irreparably destroying the inner ear. If any hearing does remain in the affected ear, the deafness doesn't become progressive.

There is no specific treatment for mumps other than painkillers and fluids. In the United States most children are given a combination measles, mumps, and rubella vaccination at 15 months to protect them against these diseases. The vaccination is given earlier in areas experiencing a measles epidemic.

External Blockage

Your child may also experience a hearing loss from a blockage in the ear canal, caused either by excess wax build-up or a foreign object. Blockages should be removed only by an ear specialist, since the eardrum could be damaged if the wax or object is pushed *into* the ear. Your doctor can remove the object by using a small device called an alligator forceps, or by using suction or fluids to flush out the blockage. It's important to have this taken care of because wax can be a fertile breeding ground for bacteria, fungi, yeasts, or viruses (especially if the ear is often submerged in water).

Intermittent Hearing Loss

A hearing problem that disappears and reappears from time to time may be related to allergies and chronic colds. This type of hearing loss is not easy to detect or treat, since sometimes the child appears to have normal hearing. If this is happening to your child, you should mention the problem to your doctor.

DOES YOUR CHILD HAVE A HEARING LOSS?

If your child shows at least two of any of the following behaviors, start observing her more closely to detect a hearing problem. Discuss your concerns with a teacher, and consider having a hearing specialist observe the child as well.

Medical history

Does your child have:
- History of ear infections
- Ringing/roaring in the ears
- History of disease with high fever
- Allergies or colds

- Earaches
- Measles or mumps

Hearing history

Does your child:
- Fail to respond to loud noises
- Watch others instead of listening to the teacher
- Constantly turn up the TV volume
- Fail to respond to instructions from someone he can't see
- Have problems locating the source of sound
- Have trouble paying attention

Speech history

Does your child:
- Constantly ask "Huh?" or "What?" or ask you to repeat things
- Have problems putting words together
- Speak infrequently
- Articulate poorly
- Have problems modulating speech volume
- Speak many words that can't be understood
- Have a nasal or oddly pitched voice

Behavior history

Does your child:
- Get easily frustrated
- Not seem to realize she's making noise
- Not become quiet at appropriate times
- Grab others to get their attention
- Breathe with his mouth open
- Seem restless
- Have a short attention span
- Play alone often

Hereditary Causes of Deafness

Not surprisingly, deafness may be caused by a wide range of inherited abnormalities. Most causes of genetic deafness are congenital (present at birth) and unchanging, and are responsible for about half of all types of deafness in children. There are about 200 different versions of genetic hearing problems, ranging in degree from mild to profound. A large percentage that occur at birth or during the first few years of life are hereditary, as are many kinds of progressive hearing losses that occur later in life. Although some kinds of hearing loss are associated with other medical problems, most types of genetic hearing loss do not involve other types of physical changes.

The ability to hear is one of many different physical traits that are handed down in families. There are several ways that genes can influence the child's ability to hear. Each person has 23 pairs of chromosomes, tiny rod-shaped structures made up of deoxyribonucleic acid (DNA), half inherited from the mother and half from the father. Inside each chromosome are thousands of genes, each one carrying the genetic building blocks for everything from the color of your hair to the size of your bones. These genes also govern the way in which the ear structures are formed. Any change in such a gene can cause a hearing problem.

Because chromosomes are paired, each segment in one chromosome has a corresponding segment in its partner. The genes—a chemical coding system of the actual units of inheritance—are also paired, one on each chromosome. Each gene provides information for the development and functioning of various organ systems. There are many different gene locations that affect hearing, and many different varieties of genes. Different types of deafness may involve different gene locations.

Autosomal recessive inheritance accounts for between 75 and 85 percent of all cases of hereditary deafness. Autosomes are the chromosomes other than the two sex chromosomes. Recessive genes are those that must come from both parents before a trait it controls is expressed. In a person whose deafness is caused by an autosomal recessive gene, both parents usually have normal hearing, but each carries a recessive gene for deafness. Usually there is no family history of deafness. If both parents have this recessive gene, their risk of having a child with this type of genetic deafness is one in four for every pregnancy. The odds of having a child who is *not* a carrier is also one in four. The remainder (one in two) will carry a recessive gene like both parents but will not be deaf.

About 20 percent of hereditary deafness is attributed to *autosomal dominant inheritance.* A gene is dominant if it is expressed when only one gene of the pair is present. Usually at least one parent is deaf and the deafness appears in each generation, affecting about the same number of girls and boys. The risk of having a second deaf child in this case is 50 percent. None of the hearing children will be carriers, because if they had the deafness gene they would be deaf themselves. The children of these hearing children would have no increased risk of having a deaf child. If *both* parents are deaf from the same type of autosomal dominant gene, they would have a 75 percent chance of having a deaf child with *each* pregnancy. With this type of deafness, there is often so much variety in the severity of the problem that it can be difficult to be sure of the pattern without careful study. (For example, one person might be profoundly deaf while that person's child might only be mildly hard of hearing).

The *X-linked inheritance pattern* occurs when an abnormal gene is located on the X chromosome. Out of all the chromosome pairs in the human body, one pair determines sex: a female has two X chromosomes in this pair (an XX pattern), and a male has one X and one Y chromosome (an XY pattern). When the 46 chromosome pairs divide in making sperm, half of the resulting sperm cells will have an X, half a Y. In X-linked genetic hearing disorders, females are usually protected because most have a normal gene on their other X chromosome. But the male, having only one X, is not protected if he receives the abnormal gene. Thus, females are carriers and have a one in two chance of giving the abnormal gene to any one son (who will be deaf), or to a daughter, who will be a carrier. Affected males cannot pass the deafness on to their sons, because they give them only the Y chromosome, but all their daughters will be carriers because they receive the damaged X chromosome from their fathers. This results in a "skipped" generational pattern: one normal-hearing carrier mother may have deaf sons, but all the children of the deaf son will be apparently normal.

Someone may have a genetic hearing loss and be the only person with that problem in the family, but if there is more than one person in the family with a hearing loss, then the problem is almost always genetic. Unfortunately, geneticists cannot often predict *which* members of a family will receive the gene for a hearing problem.

Because hearing problems are so often genetic, it is common to refer a family with a deaf member to a genetic counselor or a genetic team. Such a team may include a genetic associate (a person with a master's degree in genetic counseling), a genetics physician, and sometimes a genetics nurse or social worker.

Currently no blood test can diagnose a "hearing loss gene," but a medical geneticist can often tell whether someone's hearing problem has been inherited. Genetic counseling for hearing loss always includes a detailed family history, a medical history of the deaf person, and a pregnancy history of the mother. The individual or family is then seen by the medical geneticist for a physical examination to uncover clues in the appearance that might suggest a basis for the hearing problem, including checking the head, eyes, and ears and looking for changes in the skin, hair, or kidneys.

When it is possible to determine the cause of the hearing problem and how a gene has passed through the family, the team meets with the individual or the family and explains how the hearing loss was inherited and what the implications and possibilities are for future generations.

A number of diseases can be passed down in families that will result in hearing loss, including Paget's disease, Alport's disease, and Cogan's, Penred's, Usher's, and Waardenburg's syndromes.

Diagnosing Infants

What happens if you need to test the hearing of a newborn, who can't be expected to participate in a screening test?

Since early detection is essential so that intervention can begin immediately, medical technology has come up with a way of detecting the *brain's* response to sound that doesn't require any participation on the part of the child. Because it would be too expensive to test every newborn in order to locate the few who have a hearing problem, the screening process is usually done only with infants determined to be at "high risk." This is determined by a number of factors, including:

- A family history of hearing loss or genetic problems associated with deafness
- Blood incompatibility between mother and child
- The use of ototoxic drugs during pregnancy (especially streptomycin and kanamycin)
- Unusual bleeding during the first trimester of pregnancy
- Any problem requiring admission to the newborn intensive-care unit
- Low APGAR rating (a well-baby assessment that tests breathing, heartrate, color, muscle tone, and motor reactions)
- Maternal infection (such as herpes or cytomegalovirus during pregnancy)
- Premature delivery, fetal distress, prolonged labor, difficult delivery, or birth injury
- Infant apnea, jaundice, multiple anomalies (whatever the cause)

If a child has one or more of these factors, physicians will recommend an *auditory brainstem response test* (ABR). This hearing test measures brain-wave activity in response to sound.

As nerve impulses pass through the lower levels of your baby's brain from the auditory nerve on their way to higher brain centers, they make connections in the brainstem near the base of the skull. The ABR tests this electrical activity. It can determine how well certain portions of the infant's auditory system in the brain responds to a presented tone or beep. This test can also be used to diagnose auditory disorders; it is also useful in confirming nonorganic, or psychogenic hearing loss. It can be performed on individuals of any age.

This painless test begins with a brief click or tone pip sent into the ear. A computer analyzes the variations in the electrical signals recorded from the scalp to see if brain activity changes in response to these signals. By repeating the tones over and over and averaging the brain's response by computer, one can get a clear picture of the brain's response minus random background electrical activity in the brain. This way it's possible to establish auditory thresholds that are very similar to what could be obtained in conventional hearing tests.

Of course, the ABR can determine only whether or not the auditory signals are getting to the brain; it can't truly test whether an infant is actually *hearing* recognizable sounds.

GENETIC SERVICES CENTER OF THE GALLAUDET RESEARCH INSTITUTE

This center was established by the institute in 1984 to explore the more than 200 known genetic forms of hearing problems as well as certain other kinds of deafness acquired through environmental means. The primary function of this center is to provide genetic evaluations and counseling sessions to help deaf people and their families understand the causes and effects of hearing loss. Staffers also consult with and train audiologists, geneticists, parents, consumers, and the medical community.

FOR MORE INFORMATION ABOUT
GENETICS AND DEAFNESS

Many universities and hospitals have clinical genetic services. Ask your doctor or local health department for a list of genetic-service providers. Or contact one of these national groups:

American Society of Human Genetics
American Board of Medical Genetics
9650 Rockville Pike
Bethesda, MD 20814
(301) 571-1825

Genetic Services Center
Gallaudet University
800 Florida Ave. NE
Washington, DC 20002
(202) 651-5258 (voice/TDD)
(800) 451-8834 xt. 5258 (voice/TDD)

March of Dimes Birth Defects Foundation
Professional Education
1275 Mamaroneck Ave.
White Plains, NY 10605
(914) 428-7100

National Research Register for Hereditary Hearing Loss
Boys Town National Research Hospital
555 30th St.
Omaha, NE 68154
(402) 498-6631 (voice/TDD)

National Society of Genetic Counselors
233 Canterbury Dr.
Wallingford, PA 19086
(215) 872-7608

NATIONAL RESEARCH REGISTER
FOR HEREDITARY HEARING LOSS

This clearinghouse is dedicated to helping people interested in research on hereditary hearing loss. The register informs participating families of new research projects applicable to them and updates all families on the progress of ongoing research through its newsletter. Contact:

National Research Register for Hereditary Hearing Loss
Boys Town National Research Hospital
555 30th St.
Omaha, NE 68154
(402) 498-6631 (voice/TDD)

4

Hearing Loss in Adulthood

Aging and Deafness

More than ten million Americans have presbycusis, a type of sensorineural hearing loss that comes with age ("presby" meaning *old* and "cusis" meaning *hearing*). But having a problem with hearing as you get older doesn't really mean you have an ear *disease*—presbycusis is not medically dangerous, nor is it a symptom of senility. It's simply a function of age. If we all lived long enough, we'd all eventually develop presbycusis. Adults deafened later in life make up the vast majority of the elderly with hearing problems.

Surprisingly, by the time most men and women reach age 30, their hearing already has declined to the point that they can't hear frequencies above 15,000 cycles per second. By age 50 that drops to 12,000; at this point most people report some loss of the ability to hear everyday conversations. By age 60 most people can't hear frequencies above 10,000 cps, and at 70 it drops to no more than 6,000 cycles—well below the upper limit of everyday speech.

As you age, you start to experience changes in the hair cells within the cochlea, or the nerves attached to it, so that sound signals can't be transmitted as efficiently. Studies have shown that as you age, you lose nerve cells in the base of the cochlea where high-frequency sounds are perceived. But researchers don't know whether this degeneration is primarily due to aging or is caused by a decrease in the ability to hear specific frequencies affecting those cells.

Of course, presbycusis is not caused solely by physiological changes related to age. An older person's hearing loss may be the result simply of wax build-up in the ear or of damage to the inner ear from infection, disease, or injury. In fact, some experts believe that excessive noise accounts for more hearing loss in old age than all other factors combined.

Each person experiences the development of presbycusis differently. You may hear sounds less clearly and tones (especially high frequencies) less audibly. People with presbycusis often have trouble understanding speech, particularly in the presence of background noise. There is usually a slow decline in hearing ability, beginning with high-pitched sounds, then a loss of hearing in the middle frequencies, followed by the lowest. Because normal speech spans all these frequencies, the ability to understand conversation may vary according to the extent of the presbycusis.

Perhaps you have noticed that you have a harder time understanding conversations with women or children (whose voices are of a higher frequency). Or you may find you have a hard time understanding conversation in a group. "I found that I could hear one-on-one conversations with no problem," reports Robert, a 55-year-old electrical engineer. "But in a crowd it's much more difficult to hear. I also find that I can have problems locating where sounds are coming from. If three or four phones are ringing in our office area at the same time, I can't tell exactly *whose* phone it is that needs to be answered."

If you have started to notice hearing loss, you should immediately see an otologist (a specialist in diseases of the ear) or an otolaryngologist (a specialist in diseases of the ear, nose, and throat), and an audiologist (a professional who assesses hearing loss and provides auditory training). Unfortunately, most people with presbycusis wait an average of five years before consulting anyone.

Although hearing aids can help most people, not everyone will benefit from them. An aid should not be prescribed or fitted before an examination and hearing test are given.

Services for Older Americans

Senior citizens who begin to experience hearing loss may find help from a group called Self Help for Hard of Hearing People (SHHH), which is primarily interested in meeting the needs of people deafened later in life. Founded in the early 1980s by a former senior officer in the Central Intelligence Agency, the group stresses self-assertiveness and advocacy.

Other special services for senior citizens with hearing problems include a special department devoted to the concerns of late-deafened adults of the Alexander Graham Bell Association for the Deaf.

WARNING SIGNS OF AGE-RELATED HEARING LOSS

As you get older, you're more likely to notice a hearing problem. Here are some signs that a problem may exist. Do you:
- Have a history of ear infections
- Experience tinnitus (ringing of the ear)
- Talk louder than you used to do
- Increase the TV or radio volume
- Feel that others are mumbling
- Confuse words with similar sounds
- Have trouble hearing high-pitched sounds
- Have trouble hearing soft sounds

GROUPS FOR LATE-DEAFENED ADULTS

SHHH
7800 Wisconsin Ave.
Bethesda, MD 20814
(301) 657-2248 (voice)
(301) 657-2249 (TDD)

Alexander Graham Bell Association for the Deaf
Oral Deaf Adults Section
3417 Volta Place NW
Washington, DC 20007
(202) 337-5220 (voice/TD)

Ear Diseases

In addition to childhood disease, a number of ear diseases can result in hearing loss later in life. Among these are auditory neuritis, cholesteatoma, labyrinthitis, mastoiditis, and otosclerosis.

Auditory Neuritis

Neuritis—the inflammation of the auditory nerve—can follow infections such as scarlet or typhoid fever or any other infection with a high fever. You may notice a hearing loss immediately, although deafness usually progresses over several days or weeks. This gradual development of inflammation can cause a sensorineural deafness very much like the hearing loss that appears in old age, but it occurs much earlier in life and is usually attributed to loss of oxygen, anemia, viruses, or labyrinthitis (inflammation of the fluid-filled chambers of the inner ear).

Cholesteatoma

This chronic middle-ear inflammatory disease is a rare, serious condition in which skin cells and debris collect inside the middle ear. It usually happens when the eardrum bursts following a middle-ear infection. Cholesteatomas may rarely be present at birth, where they appear anywhere in the temporal bone. A cholesteatoma that appears later in life may be caused by a persistent narrowing of the eustachian tube that eventually pulls the upper part of the eardrum back and forms a sac in the middle ear. This type of cholesteatoma also may result from a tiny hole in the eardrum that allows skin cells of the external ear canal to move into the middle ear.

Untreated, a cholesteatoma may grow and damage the small bones in the middle ear and the surrounding bone structures, causing a conductive or a mixed hearing loss. Although a cholesteatoma is benign and will not spread to other sites in your body, it could lead to serious complications such as a secondary infection, labyrinthitis, meningitis, or a brain abscess.

Therefore, it must be removed either through the eardrum or by a mastoidectomy (removal of the mastoid bone behind the ear, together with the cholesteatoma). Repeat operations may be required, because the cyst can grow back. The operation may also require rebuilding the bones of the middle ear to restore hearing. Ear bone transplants or artificial devices may be used to reconstruct the bones.

Labyrinthitis

This is an inflammation of the labyrinth, the fluid-filled maze of inner ear chambers that sense balance. It can cause nausea, vomiting, tinnitus, vertigo, and deafness. Also called *otitis interna*, it is almost always caused by either a bacterial or viral infection that enters the inner ear from the middle ear. Physicians are concerned about this infection primarily because it might spread to the meninges (outer covering of the brain).

Bacterial labyrinthitis may be caused by mastoiditis or an untreated acute or chronic ear infection, especially if a cholesteatoma (infected skin debris) has developed. The bacteria enters the inner ear through the eroded labyrinthine capsule. Infection may also reach the inner ear from a head injury or through the bloodstream from elsewhere in the body. It can occur from contamination during certain ear operations. This type of labyrinthitis requires immediate treatment with antibiotics in order to prevent the spread of infection that might lead to meningitis or profound sensorineural hearing loss, violent vertigo, and total deafness.

Viral labyrinthitis is usually transmitted through the bloodstream and attacks the inner ear during illnesses like measles, mumps, chickenpox, shingles, or flu. With this type of sensorineural hearing loss, onset is sudden and causes a severe or profound hearing problem. Viral labyrinthitis will eventually fade away on its own, although symptoms can be relieved with antihistamines.

A third type of labyrinthitis, more common in children, is known as *meningeal labyrinthitis.* It is caused by an organism transmitted to the cochlea via the internal auditory meatus or cochlear duct. *Syphilitic labyrinthitis* is usually caused by congenital syphilis and results in a sudden, sensorineural hearing loss or a sudden increasing fluctuation of sensorineural hearing loss. Acquired syphilitic labyrinthitis is rare.

Mastoiditis

This inflammation of the mastoid bone (the bone behind your ear) is caused by a spreading infection from the middle ear to the antrum (cavity in the mastoid bone) and from there to the air cells in the bone. The result is severe pain, swelling, and tenderness behind and inside the ear, together with a fever, creamy discharge, and progressive hearing loss. The real danger is that infection may spread *inside* the skull, causing meningitis, a brain abscess, or a stroke. The infection could also spread outward, damaging the facial nerve and paralyzing the facial muscles.

Mastoiditis has become uncommon since the use of antibiotic drugs for the treatment of ear infections. Because it can be difficult to drain the infected material from the mastoid cells, it's not easy to cure this infection. High-dose antibiotic treatment for several weeks will usually clear up the problem, but a mastoidectomy (removal of the infected air cells within the mastoid bone) may be needed if it doesn't.

Menière's Disease

Menière's disease affects more than a million Americans and can be extremely incapacitating due to dizziness and hearing loss. It was first described by the French physician Prosper Menière in 1861, and the disease's most debilitating symptom is dizziness, which can make you feel that either you, or your surroundings, are spinning. This occurs together with hearing loss, nausea and vomiting, tinnitus, and fullness or pressure within the ear. Symptoms may last from a few minutes to eight hours or more, and can be profoundly disturbing. The attacks of vertigo may occur every so often every few weeks.

Although the most common form of the disease causes vertigo, hearing loss, and tinnitus, *cochlear Menière's disease* is characterized by tinnitus *without* vertigo. *Vestibular Menière's disease* causes vertigo without hearing loss.

Menière's disease tends to come and go, but the vertigo usually gets progressively worse until it peaks after several years; symptoms will then become less severe until the vertigo finally disappears. By this time, however, the patient is usually severely deaf. Normally, only one ear is affected, and the sensorineural hearing loss may get worse and worse over the years, although a few people have experienced problems in both ears. Hearing loss may vary from one person to the next, and the problem may fluctuate at first. It may start with low frequencies and then involve higher frequencies, eventually becoming permanent. A hearing test can usually reveal loudness recruitment and poor speech discrimination.

While the exact cause of Menière's disease is unknown, researchers believe the problem is related to an unexplained swelling that causes an accumulation of fluid in the inner ear, damaging delicate nerve endings. One of the strangest things about the disorder is its unpredictability; remissions come and go, lasting anywhere from six months to six years. Some researchers think Menière's disease is caused by a defect in the way the body handles carbohydrates, leading to the overproduction of insulin as a way of overcompensating, but its source remains uncertain.

Although drugs may help prevent attacks, they are usually better at easing symptoms once an attack is underway. Atropine or scopolamine can ease nausea and vomiting, and antihistamines may relieve vertigo. Barbiturates may be used for general sedation. Studies at the House Ear Institute in California, a well-known center for research and treatment of hearing disorders, found a wide range of potential links to the disorder. Among patients they studied, allergies, endocrine problems, and trauma were found in about half of the cases. Treating the separate conditions brought about improvement in about half the cases, whereas others with the same apparent conditions did not respond.

Researchers at the institute found that by severely restricting diet some patients may find their symptoms subside and hearing increase by as much as 20 dB. But the diet restrictions were severe, and subjects had to eliminate a wide range of foods from their menu: wheat, flour, eggs, chocolate, corn, and mayonnaise. Some patients at the institute who temporarily disregarded the diet restrictions noticed an immediate return of symptoms. For Menière's patients who have abnormal insulin levels and/or impaired glucose tolerance, scientists recommend six small meals of low-carbohydrate, low-cholesterol food.

If vertigo becomes truly disruptive, there are several surgical options. Vertigo is often caused by excess fluid in the inner ear, raising pressure within the ear and disturbing the delicate balance system of the body that is centered in that area. By surgically placing a shunt to drain away excess fluid, surgeons can sometimes ease the feeling of vertigo.

Other treatments vary. Some doctors recommend lifestyle changes, including reduced stress, no cigarettes or alcohol, regular exercise, and a different diet (in addition to the above restrictions, less salt and more low-fat foods).

Otosclerosis

This disorder occurs when an overgrowth of spongy bone immobilizes the stapes (the innermost bone of the middle ear), preventing sound vibrations from passing to the inner ear and resulting in conductive hearing loss. In most cases both ears are affected. It is caused by the absorption of bone followed by the production of new, loose, spongy bone. Eventually this soft bone will harden and become as dense as surrounding bone.

While the problem can occur anywhere on the temporal bone, it usually begins in front of the oval window, gradually spreading to the oval window and then the footplate of the stapes. In time this will imbed the stapes to the surrounding tissue, restricting stapedial movement. In addition, otosclerosis can affect the cochlea, causing a sensorineural hearing loss.

The disease, which begins in early adulthood (between age 15 and 35), is the most frequent cause of middle-ear hearing loss in young adults and affects about one in every 200 people. It tends to run in families and is more common in women than in men, in whites than in blacks, Native Americans, or Asians. It often occurs during pregnancy.

People with otosclerosis tend to speak softly and hear muffled sound more clearly when there is background noise. Hearing loss progresses slowly over a period of ten to fifteen years, often accompanied by tinnitus and sometimes by vertigo. The rate of hearing loss may increase during pregnancy. Eventually there may be some sensorineural hearing loss caused by damage spreading to the inner ear, which makes high tones hard to hear. Hearing tests can uncover otosclerosis, showing a conductive hearing loss greater in lower frequencies.

Hearing aids can greatly help, although the conductive deafness can only be cured by a stapedectomy, an operation in which the stapes, or stirrup, is replaced with an artificial substitute. After surgery, there may be some dizziness, which usually disappears. Hearing usually returns fairly quickly; occasionally a blood clot will appear in the middle ear, which can block sound conduction. These usually break up within a few weeks.

Unfortunately, there is also some small risk to this procedure. Though the operation can help most people, between one and two percent lose all hearing in the ear. This is the reason people with otosclerosis in both ears often choose to undergo surgery for only one ear at a time, waiting at least a year between operations. Once the inner ear is damaged, a stapedectomy may not help the problem.

Other Diseases Related to Hearing Loss

AIDS

Infection with the human immunodeficiency virus (HIV) can result in acquired immune deficiency syndrome (AIDS) or AIDS-related complex. Both AIDS and ARC are associated with neurological complications that include hearing loss; an estimated 75 percent of adult AIDS patients and 50 percent of ARC patients have abnormalities of the hearing system.

Why this happens is unknown, although direct infection of the nervous system by HIV is well documented. Hearing disorders in AIDS could be caused directly by HIV infection of the cochlea or the central auditory system. On the other hand, many AIDS complications are caused by opportunistic infections rather than the HIV itself. The most common of these infections (cytomegalovirus, or CMV) is known to damage the hearing system in congenital cases of AIDS. More than 90 percent of AIDS patients have cytomegalovirus.

Lyme Disease

Spread by ticks or other insects, Lyme disease can cause hearing loss in addition to a host of other symptoms. In the first stage of the disease, as many as 80 percent of victims will exhibit a red rash that looks like a bull's eye, surrounding the bite site and enlarging gradually over a few weeks. Any rash that is at least two inches in diameter should be considered evidence of Lyme disease. This rash can appear anywhere between three and 32 days after the bite and may be followed by intermittent flu-like symptoms. In the second stage of the disease, between 15 and 20 percent of victims experience a hearing loss, together with migraine-like headaches and painful arthritis. The hearing loss means that the infection has moved into the central nervous system, which also may lead to facial numbness, pain and weakness in arms and legs, memory loss, stiff neck, and severe fatigue.

Diabetes

This metabolic disorder causes a decrease or absence of insulin, the hormone responsible for the absorption of glucose into cells, where it's used for energy. Because diabetes tends to break down blood vessels and peripheral nerves, it can interfere with blood supply to the ear and the internal auditory canal. This can result in a breakdown of cochlear and vestibular nerves and cause a sensorineural hearing loss.

Kidney Disease

Kidney disease requiring renal dialysis and transplantation often results in a type of sensorineural hearing loss that can be caused by a number of factors, including electrolyte imbalance, inadequate dialysis, or drug toxicity. These factors can affect the components of the inner-ear fluid and alter the normal function of the cochlea.

Syphilis

The inner-ear hearing loss that occurs among adults who contract syphilis tends to appear more slowly than it does in children with congenital syphilis, as either a hearing loss or a fluctuation in intensity. Treatment with penicillin and steroids is usually given for some months; if hearing improves, the steroids may be continued indefinitely to stave off a recurrent hearing loss.

Injury and Hearing Loss

Your hearing can be affected by a head injury that can either damage the delicate hearing mechanism or the brain itself. Although the skull is designed to protect the brain and delicate internal structures such as the inner ear, severe head injury can cause both a sensorineural and conductive deafness in one or both ears. Sensorineural deafness from a severe head injury can be associated with a fracture of the temporal bones (which house the structure of the middle and inner ears). This completely destroys the hearing and balance mechanism on the affected side. This type of deafness is usually permanent, although the dizziness that can accompany it will usually fade away over a period of several weeks. The unsteadiness and swaying toward the affected side may also subside after a few months.

It's also possible to have hearing loss after a head injury that isn't severe enough to fracture the temporal bone, especially from a blow to the back or side of the head. Deafness from this type of injury is usually similar to that caused by excess noise. An injury like this also often causes dizziness, which is made worse when you change the position of your head. Although there may be hearing loss on the side of the injury, there also may be a mild hearing loss on the opposite side, due to a concussion of the inner ear.

Conductive deafness after injury is caused by blood pooling in the middle ear and external ear canal; occasionally the ossicular chain (hammer, anvil, and stirrup) is disrupted, and the eardrum is ruptured. As the blood is absorbed and the eardrum heals, hearing usually returns to its pre-injury level. Occasionally conductive deafness after a head injury can be permanent, but the maximum degree of hearing loss is usually no more than 60 dB. This means that if speech is loud enough, you can not only hear but understand what is being said. Surgery also can sometimes restore hearing in this type of injury.

Hearing loss as a result of such damage to the middle ear can sometimes be corrected; a ruptured eardrum can heal itself in time, and the small bones of the ear may be repaired or replaced. Using the modern technique of microsurgery, ear specialists can repair or rebuild an eardrum in many cases. Using a technique called *myringoplasty*, surgeons can close a hole in the eardrum using a tissue graft from elsewhere in the body.

Normally permanent hearing loss is mild, although the loss may be greater if the ear is very sensitive or the noise was quite loud. Because there is almost always some amount of temporary hearing loss after an acoustic trauma, some time must pass before the amount of permanent damage can be measured.

Drugs and Deafness

A person can develop a hearing problem after using certain drugs or chemicals that affect hearing and balance by interfering with the function of the inner ear. The negative effect of some ototoxic drugs are increased when taken in combination with other drugs or when taken for long periods of time. Often tinnitus (ringing in the ear) is the first symptom, although some damage can occur before any symptoms appear. The developing fetus is particularly susceptible to these drugs.

A number of factors place some people at higher risk when taking ototoxic drugs, including age, earlier ear infections, prior sensorineural hearing loss, impaired kidney or liver function, extreme drug sensitivity, or simultaneous use of loop diuretics or drugs that are toxic to the kidneys.

The hallmark warning sign of imminent ear damage is tinnitus, so if you're taking any of the following drugs and you experience ringing in your ears, you should immediately consult the doctor who prescribed the medication.

Antibiotics

A few kinds of powerful antibiotics, taken to fight a life-threatening infection, may be associated with hearing loss. Though some of these drugs cause a permanent hearing loss, the law requires that you be told if one of these ototoxic drugs is being prescribed.

The most common class of ototoxic antibiotics is the aminoglycosides, which appear to cause hearing problems when dosage is continued for more than ten days. (The exception to this is streptomycin, which can cause a hearing loss within five days.) Any patient treated for longer than this time should undergo cochlear and vestibular testing before, during, and after therapy. Examples of the aminoglycosides include amikacin, gentamicin, kanamycin, neomycin, and streptomycin.

Neomycin is considered to be the most toxic of all drugs to the cochlea, and damage may result in hearing loss that continues irreversibly even after treatment is stopped. Warning signs may include tinnitus or impaired balance, but these symptoms don't always occur.

Other types of antibiotics, including erythromycin and viomycin, also can cause hearing loss. However, all known cases of erythromycin ototoxicity have been reversed once the drug has been discontinued, and only large doses (more than four grams per day) have been associated with erythromycin toxicity. Viomycin, on the other hand, can cause permanent hearing loss.

Loop Diuretics

Use of loop diuretics (anti–water-retention drugs) should be avoided in premature infants and in those receiving aminoglycoside antibiotics. While permanent hearing loss is possible, most of the time the loss, vertigo, and tinnitus is reversible within 30 minutes and a day after medication is stopped. Examples of these drugs include furosemide (rapid IV administration increases chances of hearing problems), ethacrynic acid, bumetanide, and indapamide.

Aspirin and Salicylates

High doses of salicylates (such as about 10 pills of aspirin or drugs with aspirin in them per day) can cause ringing of the ears and a hearing loss of up to 40 decibels, both directly related to the amount of the drug in the bloodstream. Although many drugs can be toxic to the delicate sensory tissue of the ear and can cause permanent hearing loss, aspirin is unusual in that the inner-ear hearing loss it causes is reversible. Both hearing loss and tinnitus will disappear within one to three days after the drug is stopped. Normally, you'd have to take more than ten aspirin tablets a day before there is a danger of hearing loss, although every person's sensitivity to the drug is different. Patients who already have some degree of sensorineural hearing loss may find that aspirin can have a stronger effect on hearing at lower frequencies.

Quinine Derivatives

Quinine is the oldest drug treatment for malaria, but less than two grams a day may cause a transient tinnitus, hearing loss, vertigo, headache, nausea, or vision problems. There have been cases of permanent hearing loss and tinnitus, but usually only when high doses of the drugs were continued after symptoms appeared. Examples of these drugs include quinine, chloroquine, quinidine, and hydroxychloroquine.

Anti-Cancer Drugs

A few chemotherapy drugs such as cysplatin may also cause a hearing loss, but many patients accept the risk in an effort to cure their cancer.

Other Substances

Substances that may temporarily reduce hearing ability or increase tinnitus include alcohol, carbon monoxide, caffeine, oral contraceptives, and tobacco.

5

Noise and Hearing Loss

George, age 45, has been a master automotive technician for the past 25 years. During that time his ears have been assaulted daily by the noises common in a busy auto-repair shop: the blast of air-driven tools, the crash of metal against metal. He admits his hearing loss has been getting worse with every year he remains in the shop. Today, there are many sounds in the higher frequencies he cannot hear at all.

"I'm always very careful to wear goggles to protect my eyes," he says. "I guess I don't think so much about my ears. You just can't keep putting ear protectors on and off, and you never know when a loud noise might happen."

George is not alone. It may surprise you to learn that up to one-third of all hearing loss can be traced at least in part to the loud noises of modern life. It could be just one brief, very loud noise, such as a gunshot, or by the continuous blare of loud rock music. Did you ever wince in momentary pain at the boom of a stereo, the whine of a snowmobile, or the crack of a gun? What most people don't realize is that *any* noise loud enough to cause pain is loud enough to damage the delicate hearing mechanism within your ears.

Over the years you may have noticed that when you hear a sudden, intensely loud noise, it is often accompanied by an immediate sense of fullness or tinnitus (ringing in the ear). If the noise is loud enough, it can rupture the eardrum and disrupt the chain of tiny bones in the ear called the hammer, anvil, and stirrup. This type of injury can cause a conductive hearing loss without much accompanying nerve damage because the middle-ear damage actually protects the inner ear.

Generally, the fullness and tinnitus subside after the injury, and hearing improves, although there may be some degree of permanent hearing loss. The amount of loss depends on the intensity and duration of the noise and the sensitivity of the ear. In milder cases the hearing loss occurs only in the ear that had been closer to the loud noise.

On the other hand, listening to very loud noises for a long period of time can damage the tiny hairs deep within the ears. This type of loss is common in people who work in very loud jobs without protection or in those who listen to loud rock music. Such chronic loud noise can damage your body in other ways. Research has found that these types of loud, persistent noises can cause changes throughout the human body, not just in the ears, including peripheral blood-vessel constriction, blood-pressure and heartrate increases, balance problems, and increases in gastrointestinal activity.

Hearing loss resulting from recreational noise is becoming more and more common. Some of the activities associated with loud noise and hearing loss include trapshooting, driving or riding recreational vehicles (like snowmobiles), and listening to extremely loud music. Even the roar of a subway train can hurt your ears.

The problem is, we don't think it will ever happen to us. It did to Kathy Peck, former bass player and lead singer of an all-female punk band whose trademark was very loud music. When her band opened for Duran Duran at the Oakland Coliseum in California in 1984, Peck remembers that her ears kept ringing for days afterward. By her mid-twenties, Peck discovered she had lost more than 40 percent of her hearing because of years spent playing in front of huge speakers turned up full blast.

If you work in a noisy environment, you probably know you should be wearing hearing protectors or you could stand a good chance of damaging your hearing. But those of you who like to sit right in front of the speakers at a rock music concert, or crank up your stereo until the walls shake, are probably doing some very real damage to your inner ear, too. Even using earphones to listen to loud music from a portable radio can hurt your ears, since it conducts the teeth-rattling noise directly into the delicate mechanisms of the inner ear.

Danger Zone

How loud is too loud? Prolonged exposure to noise above 90 decibels is enough to damage the hair cells that line the cochlea of the inner ear. To give you an idea of how loud that is, imagine standing on the sidewalk in New York City at rush hour. The street noise level in that situation is about 80 decibels, which is teetering at the very edge of the "safe" range. The noise of a motorcycle or snowmobile lies between 85 and 90 dB, and most rock concerts have been clocked between 80 and 100 dB. If you stand three feet away from a jackhammer without ear protectors, you're most likely damaging your ears from the 120 dB noise level; a jet engine from 100 feet away puts out noise at 130 dB. For this reason, jet engine mechanics are at high risk for hearing loss if they work without some type of ear protectors. All military aircraft mechanics are required to wear protection.

"If you're working on a jet engine all day," says Gerry, 43, a jet airplane mechanic, "you have to wear ear protectors because you can't stand the noise. There might be 60 people working on one jet, and everyone is using air tools and noisy machinery. We didn't always wear earplugs when we worked on smaller planes outside, though. When I'd work outside all day on a smaller plane and I wouldn't wear ear plugs, my ears would be ringing by the end of the day."

This ringing that Gerry noticed serves as the ear's warning signal that your ears are at risk. Although he would recover from exposure to just one day of this noise, it could still have cost him a few hair cells within his ears. The more days that he was exposed to noise at this level, the more hair cells would die. Injured hair cells can lead to a sensorineural hearing loss because the damage affects the transference of sound within the inner ear. A hair cell once destroyed can never be regenerated.

Risky Job Environments

A number of industrial jobs produce enough noise to impair hearing. In part, this occurs because while noise above 90 dB can damage your hearing, a person can work in the presence of noise up to 120 dB before it really begins to be painful.

If you work at a job in the presence of 90 dB noise, you probably don't think that your hearing could really be damaged. You might experience a brief, slight ringing or muffling of sounds, but after a day away from the job, these symptoms probably fade away. Even in the presence of significant noise up to 120 dB, a person tested after working all day under these conditions might show a slight loss of hearing, and after a few days away from the job a retest would reveal hearing has returned to normal. This is called a *temporary threshold shift*. However, after several months of this type of exposure, hearing loss would become permanent.

At first you probably won't notice work-induced hearing loss because deficits show up first among the high frequencies, which doesn't interfere much with the understanding of speech. You might not notice a problem until your hearing loss worsens and begins to affect the middle frequencies; by that time the loss may be permanent.

If you work around noisy machinery, you should understand that if it is necessary to raise your voice to be heard by
someone less than two feet away, protective devices should be
worn. A person working in an environment this noisy should
have a hearing test once a year and always wear ear protectors—or find a different job! It's important to keep in mind
that you won't become used to working around noise; if after
some months or years the noise seems less noticeable, it is
only because you've already sustained a hearing loss.

The Occupational Health and Safety Act includes a wide
range of rules to protect workers in many dangerous occupa-
tions. An essential requirement of this act states that any
industry in which employees are exposed daily to continuous
noise levels of more than 90 dB for eight hours must either
reduce the noise, or protect the hearing of exposed workers.

Although studies indicate that continual exposure to 90 dB
noise will result in a hearing loss of about 15 dB, it does not
mean that everyone who works in this environment will have
the same loss; some workers' ears are damaged and others
remain healthy. Still others sustain a hearing loss of more
than 30 dB. This is because hearing loss is also related to the
level of noise *outside* work, which can vary a great deal.

At this time the only way to protect your ears against
damage from noise in excess of 80 dB for eight hours a day is
to wear protective ear devices such as ear plugs or earmuffs.

Noise-Control Laws

Legislation aimed at controlling public noise is certainly
not new. Julius Caesar issued an ordinance banning chariots
from the streets of Rome during the night so he could sleep
in peace. But it was not until the mid-twentieth century that
modern legislation aimed at controlling noise in public was
first enacted. In 1968, the U.S. Congress first passed noise-
control laws as part of its amendment to the Federal Aviation

OTOTOXIC JOBS

If you work in one of the following jobs, you are at risk for hearing loss. They include:

- boilermaking
- weaving
- aircraft maintenance
- blacksmithing
- riveting
- blasting
- machine manufacturing
- metalworking
- loud rock music production

In addition, you could be at risk if you work in any job involving:

- large presses
- high-pressure steam
- large wood saws
- heavy hammering (such as iron or steelworking)

Act. A year later Congress included hearing-conservation rules for plants with federal contracts.

Unusual in their inclusion of safety provisions for private enterprise, the regulations paved the way for the Occupational Health and Safety Act of 1970, which brought together a host of safety regulations in industry. Included was a section that applied the noise regulations to all workers in all industries.

The 1970 law requires industry to define areas in their plants where noise exceeds 90 dB for an eight-hour workday; each time noise level increases 5 dB, an employee's allowable exposure time is cut in half. The law notes that it's better to lower excessive noise, but if workers can't be protected by limiting the exposure or the level of the noise, the law requires they be given either protective hearing devices or annual hearing tests to identify those with progressive hearing loss.

This 1970 legislation was followed two years later by the Noise Control Act, which gave the Environmental Protection Agency power over federal regulatory action in noise control. The Labor Department maintains control over the Occupational Safety and Health Administration, and the Federal Aviation Agency retains authority over aircraft noise-regulatory action.

NOISE LEVEL LIMITS

Ear protectors must be worn in any job whose noise level tops the following limits, according to the U.S. Occupational Safety and Health administration:

Decibels	Hours
90	8
95	4
100	2
110	$1/2$
115	$1/4$

Ear Protectors

There are two basic types of ear-protecting devices: earplugs, which fit inside the ear canal, and earmuffs, which fit outside the ears like the type of earmuffs used in cold weather. Earplugs and earmuffs worn together provide the most effective protection against noise.

The most important factor in how well any device protects your hearing is the quality of the seal. How can you tell if your protector is doing the job? Try talking to yourself. Your voice should sound lower, muffled, and a bit louder than when you aren't wearing protectors, since you are hearing the sound via bone conduction inside your head. Other sounds around you should be much quieter.

Ear-protection devices have recently been assigned a noise-reduction rating (NRR) that can indicate the ability to protect you from noise. Ear protectors now on the market range from 0 to 30 NRR. For the best protection, look for those listed with a range above 20.

If you want to use earplugs to protect yourself against noise, don't buy the pre-molded kind available at drugstores (such as the ones designed for swimming). Most of the over-the-counter plugs are usually available in one size only, and people's ears are not the same size. You really need the right size earplugs to block sound adequately. To be effective in screening out excess noise, earplugs must fit snugly in the ear canal so that no air can get through. If your ears happen to be the same size as the plugs sold in the store, you might get a good fit, and you'll certainly save money over the years. The rest of us should buy custom earplugs.

Custom-fit earplugs, which are made to fit only your ears, are a good choice, especially if you have a special problem with a noisy environment or work in a high-risk profession. Custom plugs are usually sold by an audiologist or hearing aid dispenser.

In fitting the earplugs, the dealer will make an impression of the ear canal and send the dimensions to a manufacturer, where the soft rubber earplug insert is made. These plugs have an excellent NRR when new, but they shrink with age, which can be within a few months of purchase. These fitted earplugs should be used only by adults, since the ear canals of children and teenagers change rapidly. Earplugs must fit properly in order to shut out sound and must be kept clean to avoid infection. Most types give about 30 dB protection against excess noise.

What *won't* work as an earplug is dry cotton; it's almost useless in protecting against excess noise. Some types of disposable ear protectors made of a combination of cotton, wax, and other specially treated material are somewhat effective.

The new flexible foam cylinder ear protectors give excellent noise protection (up to 28 NRR) and can be a great value at less than a dollar per pair. Instead of having them fitted by a dealer, you simply compress the foam-rubber cylinders and place them in your ear canals, where they re-expand and form an extremely good seal. However, because they can't be washed, they must be regularly replaced.

Earmuffs can provide effective sound protection. Some people find that the shape of their ear canals mean they simply can't wear earplugs without pain. Others find the feeling of something plugging their ears objectionable.

Earmuffs completely cover the ear and are made of sponge material held in place by a tension headband. Earmuff protectors generally cost more than earplugs, but they are harder to lose and some believe they are more comfortable for daily wear. If you wear glasses, however, you may find that the glasses interfere with the earmuffs' seal. Earmuff protectors are commonly found in sporting-goods stores and can cost more than $20.

Take Control of Noise

If you work in a fairly noisy environment, there may be some other things you can do to modify your working area to cut down on noise instead of resorting to ear protectors. Try these suggestions:

- Place foam pads under noisy machines (printers, typewriters, meat grinders, food processors, copiers)
- Wrap noisy, large machines with insulating materials
- Mount noisy machines on rubber, not concrete
- Use the special noise-reduction plastic boxes sold for encasing computers and printers
- Make sure there are drapes and carpeting where you work

Remember that to work in the presence of constant noise can have a real effect on your ability to hear. While it may not be convenient to wear ear protectors or take extra measures to soften the noise, coping with significant hearing loss can be far more inconvenient and expensive.

TINNITUS AIDS

Ringing or buzzing in the ears (tinnitus) is caused by a number of factors, including trauma from exposure to loud noise, an ear disease, aging, or from a side effect of some drugs. In many cases there is no known cause. If this happens to you, remember that tinnitus is a symptom, not a disease. It can't physically harm you.

But how do you live with that annoying constant noise? In addition to seeing an ear specialist, try these tips:

- *Maskers.* A device that substitutes one sound for another; it can be anything from listening to a radio to make the tinnitus less obvious to purchasing a device that looks like a hearing aid but instead delivers a pleasant sound that's matched to your tinnitus pitch. You can buy these devices from an audiologist.
- *Lifestyle.* Since excessive alcohol and nicotine cause tinnitus to worsen, try cutting back on drinking and smoking.
- *Exercise.* Improving your circulation may help.
- *Stress.* Try to reduce your daily stress levels. If you find you are troubled by stress, anxiety, and insomnia, you may want to discuss antianxiety medication (such as Xanax or Valium) with your doctor.

6

Do You Need a Hearing Aid?

If you had problems seeing the sentence in this book, odds are you wouldn't think twice about getting glasses or contact lenses. But most people who start to have problems with their hearing are not nearly so willing to buy a hearing aid. Surprisingly, only about 20 percent of Americans with a hearing loss actually use an aid. In part, this is because many people equate wearing a hearing aid with getting old. Others don't really notice their hearing loss, because it happens so gradually. For still others, getting a hearing aid means admitting that a hearing loss exists, and they don't want to face those particular facts.

"My grandchildren tell me I'm losing my hearing," says Helen, 76. *"They want me to get a hearing aid. But I don't want to wear one. My friends have told me they are unpleasant to wear. I'd rather not hear than have to walk around with a hearing aid stuck in my ear."*

Buying a hearing aid just isn't as simple as going to the local mall on a one-hour stop for glasses. You need to know what kind of hearing loss you have, conductive or sensorineural. Can you hear low tones or high pitches? Do you have problems with only some words or entire conversations? What sort of environment do you need an aid for? Is background noise a problem? Do you hear poorly with one ear or both? Hearing aids come in a wide range of styles and types, requiring careful testing to make sure the aid is the best choice for your particular hearing problem. New technology has made quite a difference in the way aids compensate for hearing loss, and there are a great number of parameters to consider. The good news is that the overall quality of conventional hearing aids has vastly improved in the past five years.

You may have never thought about a hearing aid. You may have contemplated an aid and then rejected the idea. Or you may have bought an aid only to end up leaving it in a drawer when you became frustrated with using it. This is what happened to Sarah Daniels, who at age 81 finally agreed with her grandchildren to see a specialist about her hearing. After extensive testing which revealed a moderate hearing loss, she was fitted with a hearing aid. But when her grandchildren came to visit, they discovered the TV blasting and the expensive device languishing in a drawer. "I hated it," Sarah told them. "I'd rather be deaf than have to fool around with a hearing aid." Before learning about the different types of aids—and what's new on the horizon—it's a good idea to fully understand what an aid can and can't do.

Pros and Cons

A hearing aid can boost the loudness of sound, which can improve your understanding of speech. You will be able to hear high-pitched sounds, and aids may help you feel better in social situations. Moreover, the hearing aid can alert people that you do have a hearing problem, which may remind them to make a more concerted effort of communicating with you.

You still won't be able to hear very soft sounds, because if the hearing aid was set to pick up these sounds, normal speech would be far too loud for comfortable listening. Even with a perfectly working hearing aid, you will probably still have a slight hearing loss. Basically, an aid modifies the sound traveling into your ear. Once it gets there, if your brain and inner ear distort that sound, the aid can't do anything about that distortion. It can only make this distorted sound louder and help you try to figure out the noise.

One of the main problems with most hearing aids is that they amplify *all* sounds, not just the ones you want to hear. Particularly when the source of sound is far away, such as up on a stage or in a large building, environmental noise can interfere with good perception. And although a hearing aid can amplify sound, it doesn't necessarily improve the *clarity* of that sound.

Let's face it, a hearing aid is a machine. It can never duplicate the true sound that people with normal hearing experience. Some consumers say that the sound produced by a hearing aid is mechanical and artificial. And if you're in a crowded, noisy theater, your hearing aid won't screen out all that background noise—it will amplify *everything*, making it difficult for you to discriminate conversation. Furthermore, it might not help you understand the words of speakers across the room (such as in church or at a meeting).

A hearing aid won't return your hearing to normal levels, but it will help you take advantage of what hearing you have by making sounds louder and speech easier to understand for those with certain types of hearing loss.

In addition, hearing aids favor sounds in the frequency of speech, which means that sounds that lie outside this range may be altered. Remember, no matter what type of aid your audiologist recommends, it will require practice and skill to be used effectively.

FDA REGULATIONS ON HEARING AIDS

The Food and Drug Administration has established the following regulations on hearing aids to protect the health and safety of those with hearing problems. They require:

- A medical test by a licensed physician (preferably one specializing in ear diseases) within six months before the purchase of a hearing aid.
- A doctor's written assessment may be waived by the client (18 years of age or older) on signing a document to this effect. Children, however, *must* be evaluated by a physician.
- Health professionals who dispense hearing aids must refer consumers to a physician if any of eight specified ear conditions are evident: ear deformity, drainage, sudden or progressive hearing loss, dizziness, significant ear wax, foreign body, pain, or discomfort.
- A user's instruction book with every hearing aid, specifying the importance of medical evaluation, instructions for proper use, repair service information, care information, known side effects, etc.

Hearing Aids Today

Today's hearing aids are a far cry from the ear trumpet of the Victorian age. The first true hearing aid appeared in 1921 after the invention of the vacuum tube, but these devices were cumbersome units with large parts and heavy batteries. Modern hearing aid systems consist of a small microphone designed to pick up sound waves and convert them into electrical signals that are fed into an amplifier. The amplifier boosts the signal and sends it to a receiver, which converts the amplified signals back into sound and transmits them into the ear through an earmold.

If the earmold is properly fitted, it carries the amplified sound directly into the ear canal. A poorly fitting earmold, however, causes whistles and squeals and can irritate or hurt your ears. This is why custom-fitted molds are a better idea than ready-made types.

People with only a mild hearing loss may get enough improvement simply with a tiny unit that fits directly into the ear; those with more severe problems may need a larger, more powerful system. Worn on the body, they are sturdier, easier to regulate, and less subject to distortion.

Modern hearing aids do much more than amplify sound, however; they can also filter background noise, change tonal quality, and control the loudness of environmental sounds. Researchers have been able to devise smaller and smaller units that are less visible, which appeals to those who don't want others to know they wear hearing aids.

Getting an Aid

As we have seen in earlier chapters, the first step in getting a hearing aid is to have a medical exam and a hearing evaluation. In fact, most states prohibit anyone from selling a hearing aid to you before you have been examined by a physician who can rule out the possibility of a medical problem. (Waivers are permitted for those whose religious beliefs preclude physician visits.)

Hearing Aid Evaluation

Based on your tests, there are several ways for an audiologist to determine what sort of hearing aid you should have:

- *Personal judgment.* Your audiologist might ask you at what level of loudness conversation is comfortable and determine general characteristics of the appropriate aid from your answers.

- *Formulas.* Some audiologists take the results of your hearing tests and apply mathematical formulas to come up with a recommendation.

At this time an audiologist will recommend what type of hearing aid you should buy. He may make a general suggestion about certain characteristics that might help your situation, or he might have a specific recommendation complete with brand name. This variation in judgment is due to the fact that some people require specific characteristics that are available only with certain aids. On the other hand, the audiologist might have found that certain companies are more reliable or offer better repair services.

The audiologist should be willing to discuss the different types of hearing aids such as *digital, behind-the-ear, on-the-body,* and so forth. Although a dispensing audiologist can sell you an aid, you aren't under any obligation to buy it from the person who conducted your hearing evaluation.

If your audiologist does *not* sell hearing aids, she can give you a list of competent dealers in your area. You may also request such a list even if the audiologist is a dealer. Remember that you have the right to shop around, to compare prices, and to ask about what services are included.

Prices for hearing evaluations vary across the country, but most range between $35 to $125 for a hearing aid evaluation. You can expect to pay less at a university-related clinic.

After performing a hearing evaluation, an audiologist should be able to determine whether a hearing aid will help you and what type will do the most good. This is especially important since aids can be expensive—you don't want to waste time and money on the wrong one. Once you've gotten your diagnosis and hearing test, and the experts determine that you can benefit from an aid, you're ready for your first hearing aid consultation.

Who Fits an Aid?

Since a hearing aid represents quite an investment—between $500 and $4,000—it's important to find a reliable dealer who can help you choose what model will work best for you. Complaints to state licensing boards indicate some consumers have trouble locating someone to adjust or replace their hearing aid or who will refund the price of an aid when it doesn't work as they expected. A few unscrupulous dealers may try to sell you an aid with the largest profit margin rather than matching the device with your particular needs, or they may sell you an aid whether you really need one or not.

In all but three states, hearing aids must be fitted and sold only by licensed specialists, who may be called *dealers, specialists, dispensers,* or *dispensing audiologists.* While you can buy an aid through the mail, experts caution that it's not a good idea. The pattern of your hearing loss will be quite different than someone else's, and what works for them won't work for you. That's why aids sold through the mail without individual testing may be ineffective or downright harmful.

If there is no audiologist who can sell you a hearing aid in your area, you might want to have your physician recommend a hearing-aid dealer. Before audiologists moved into the dealership field, hearing aids were sold exclusively by people who were not required to have additional training in the field. Most learned the trade by apprenticing to an experienced dealer; for many years no licensure or registration was required.

Today, however, a license is required for all dealers except those in Colorado, Massachusetts, and Minnesota. Your dealer should be licensed or certified by the National Board for Certification of Hearing Instrument Sciences (look for the initials BC-HIS). In order to be licensed, a person combines study with training under a licensed professional and then must pass a state examination. As audiologists move into the hearing aid–dispensing field, state licensing exams are being designed with an emphasis on audiological education.

While some dealers call themselves audiologists, this title should be used only by those who have earned at least a master's degree in audiology. If you're wondering about a dealer's reputation, you can check with your local Better Business Bureau, the state attorney general's office, or the licensing board in your state for records of past consumer complaints.

Shop Around

Odds are if you go to a dealer who offers only one brand of hearing aid, you'll end up paying more than you need to spend. By shopping around, you may be able to save several hundred dollars. It's common practice for dealers and audiologists to pool their resources and form a buying group, obtaining hearing aids from private manufacturers and selling them under a private label. These labels can save you up to half off the cost, but only if you buy from a dealer who passes along the savings. And remember that even a dealer who offers several brands may push one over another because of manufacturer incentives.

This is why it's a good idea to get a copy of your hearing-test results (you may have to pay extra for this) and get price quotes from several dealers before you buy a hearing aid. If you have your records, you can take your test results to other audiologists or dealers for a second opinion on the best type of hearing aid for you.

Do a little research. The Veterans Administration tests different brands of aids every year to determine where to buy its aids. Though the list is not comprehensive, it's safe to assume that any aid the VA considers satisfactory should be acceptable. (Of course, if an aid you're interested in *isn't* on the list, it could mean that it simply hasn't yet been tested by the VA.) For a copy of the VA test results, request the "Hearing Aids" publication #1B-11/78A from the Department of Veterans Affairs, Forms and Publications Dept., 6307 Gravel Ave., Alexandria, VA 22310.

WHAT TO LOOK FOR WHEN BUYING A HEARING AID

- Look for a dealer who offers a wide variety of aids; avoid anyone with just one type or brand.
- Determine exactly what's included in the price (including initial testing, the aid, the fitting, and follow-up visits).
- Look for a dealer who offers follow-up care.
- Make sure your dealer can service what he sells; many will allow you to use a "loaner" aid while yours is being repaired.
- Find out about service and a warranty when you buy the aid.
- Make sure you have a 30-day trial period to try out the hearing aid (this is required by law in some states) so that you can return the aid within that time for a full refund if it doesn't sufficiently improve your hearing.
- Watch out for "nonrefundable fees" (sometimes called "restocking fee" or "dispensing fee" in the fine print of your contract). Only the cost of testing and the price of a part that must be custom-fitted to your own ear should be nonrefundable.

The Process Begins

Once you've selected a hearing aid dispenser/dealer, the specialist will make an impression of your ears using a putty-like material, from which a personalized earmold will be created. It's the dealer's job to make sure the aid fits properly, so feel free to discuss how it feels.

The dealer also should help you:

- Schedule several visits to help you find the right hearing aid, teach you how to use it, and keep it in good working order

- Learn how to put the aid on, adjust the controls, and take it off
- Outline a schedule for wearing the aid
- Teach you how to maintain the device
- Give you suggestions on getting used to your hearing aid
- Discuss new hearing aid models and the conditions in which each type can be used
- Be willing to service the aid
- Provide information about what to do if you develop a sensitivity to the earmold (some people are allergic to the materials used to manufacture the device)

Once you have your hearing aid, make an appointment to return to the dealer/dispenser in about three weeks to try on the earmold and hearing aid. Adjustments will be made at this time. Within several weeks you should return again to the dealer's office to have the aid checked and to discuss your progress in dealing with wearing it. Since 40 percent of all hearing aids require some modification or adjustment to get

---

BASIC HEARING AID PACKAGE

Since hearing aids are not inexpensive—and are often not covered by insurance—you'll want to make sure you get good value for your money. The following services should be included in the total price quote for a hearing aid:
- Cost of the hearing aid
- Cost of the earmold(s)
- Battery pack
- Adjustments to the hearing aid or earmold
- Counseling and orientation
- Return visits (at least two)
- Warranty (at least one year)

the best results, it is certainly not unusual if you feel the need to return for a check-up. Within the first month after you purchase a hearing aid, make an appointment for a full hearing examination to determine if the aid is functioning properly.

HEARING AID COSTS

Price	Device
$500–750	Good choice for those with mild to moderate hearing loss. This price should cover a decent behind-the-ear aid with 30-day follow-up, six-month check-up, and one-year warranty; the higher cost may buy an in-the-ear aid.
$700–1,000	Behind-the-ear aid with options, or in-the-ear or canal aid. Most of these aids should have automatic signal processing (K-amp circuitry, for example).
$1,000–1,200	Conventional aid with options; lower-end digital aid. Consider a digital if you have moderate to severe loss, if conventional aids don't help, or if you change listening environments.
$1,200–up	Behind-the-ear or in-the-ear digitally programmed aid.

These prices are estimate ranges that vary depending on the part of the country where you live. Prices may vary widely even in the same geographical location.

PAYING FOR HEARING AIDS

If you think you might have trouble paying for a hearing aid, the following sources may be able to help. Check the appendix for addresses for these groups:

- Local service clubs (Lion's Club, Kiwanis Club, SERTOMA, Optimists Club, Quota International Club)
- Local chapter of United Way
- Local department of social services
- Organizations serving deaf or hard-of-hearing people
- Medicaid (offers limited reimbursement)
- Vocational rehabilitation agency
- State agency on aging
- State office/commission on deafness
- Veterans Administration (for veterans)
- Easter Seals Society
- Hear Now (runs a bank for donated aids)

Types of Hearing Aids

Once it's been determined that a hearing aid may be able to improve your hearing, you'll be faced with a choice of several different types of aids. On the one hand, most hearing aids are fairly simple in theory—a microphone, amplifier, and speaker, powered by a battery. But as technology has improved, hearing aids have become smaller and smaller, so it's now possible to buy a device tiny enough to fit entirely inside your ear, barely visible from the outside.

Depending on the style of hearing aid you buy, you might be able to add a number of features so you can filter or block background noise, minimize feedback, lower sound in noisy settings, and boost your power when needed. Of course, you need to keep in mind that no matter how fancy your aid is, if it increases the sound of speech it's bound to amplify some background noise as well.

HEARING AID GLOSSARY

There are four main characteristics when talking about hearing aids:

- *Gain:* This is a measure of the power of your hearing aid and how much it amplifies sound.
- *Frequency range:* This explains how much power your hearing aid has in certain range of pitches and how far your aid can amplify the high and low pitches.
- *Maximum power output:* A measure of the loudest sound the hearing aid can produce; this can act as a safety valve against damage to your ear from sudden loud noises.
- *Distortion:* This is a measure of how well the hearing aid reproduces sound. Any electronic device (such as your TV or radio) distorts sound to some degree.

Although some exciting strides have been made in the hearing aid industry, it's still possible to divide the devices into one of four categories: digital, behind-the-ear, in-the-ear, and in-the-canal.

Digital Aids

These are the new kids on the hearing aid block—an exciting advance in technology that may offer real improvement to those who are beginning to lose their hearing.

As we've seen, one of the biggest complaints many people have with hearing aids is that they tend to amplify environmental noise without significantly improving the ability to hear other individuals. This is because most people have hearing loss for high-frequency sounds of speech, which tend to be soft. If you wear a conventional hearing aid, it will amplify the din of a New Year's Eve party beyond endurance while not letting you hear the person next to you offer you more bean dip.

The solution may be a digital aid. These sophisticated and very expensive hearing aids borrow computer technology to allow you to tailor an aid to your specific hearing loss pattern. Unlike most modern aids, these state-of-the-art devices contain miniature computer chips that can selectively boost certain frequencies while leaving others alone. Wearing such an

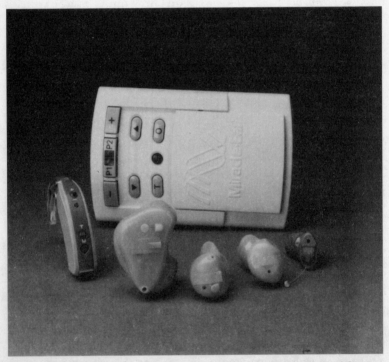

Some of the newest hearing aids are digitally programmable and feature a remote control device (in rear) for adjusting tone and volume. These aids can be adjusted to perform well in different settings, from a noisy cocktail party to a quiet restaurant. From left, the programmable aids include the behind-the-ear, contour aid, semi-contour, canal aid, and completely in-the-canal aid. (Courtesy Dahlberg, Inc.)

aid to that same New Year's Eve party, you could screen out the excess background noise while focusing in on the person with the dip.

The aid is programmed by the dealer/dispenser to amplify different frequencies to different degrees to fit your hearing loss pattern. Though standard hearing aids have only limited capacity to make adjustments, the new digital models permit much finer tuning. Several models also have programmable memories that allow you to choose different settings depending on how noisy the situation, so you could switch programs as you walk from a quiet park to a downtown subway to normal at-home relaxing.

This digital aid is the first device that is adaptable to the individualized needs of the wearer. This is important, since people with hearing loss don't all experience the same problems with the same loss in frequency and decibel levels.

Up until now modern aids mimicked the sound waves of normal hearing via electrical signals. Digital hearing aids translates sound into electrical impulses that can be captured in precise computer code and manipulated just like any other software. This should make it easier to filter out background noise and provide truer sound. It's particularly exciting since one of the most difficult situations for people with hearing aids is to communicate in a crowded room with lots of other voices and background noise.

There are several different types of digital aids. One type divides the sound spectrum into a number of separate bands; amplification for each band is programmed to match your pattern of hearing loss. A more expensive digital aid (more than $2,000) uses only two frequency bands, but within each band the aid can be adjusted to give loud sounds less amplification than soft ones.

While experts still aren't sure if the digital devices will be the answer for everyone, the potential pool of consumers is enormous—as many as 25 million hard-of-hearing people may be able to make use of the technology. If you have a moderate to severe hearing loss and you travel from one kind of

DIGITAL PROGRAMMABLE HEARING AIDS

Here is a partial list of manufacturers of digital programmable hearing aids who can provide you more detailed information about their products.

Bausch & Lomb
Hearing System Division
7555 Market Place Dr.
Eden Prairie, MN 55344
(800) 331-5321
MODEL NAME: Quantum

GN Danavox, Inc.
5600 Rowland Rd., Ste. 150
Minnetonka, MN 55343
(800) 432-7835
MODEL NAME: 143 Pro

Ensoniq Corp.
155 Great Valley Pkwy.
Malvern, PA 19355
(800) 942-0096
MODEL NAME: Sound Selector

Maico Hearing Instruments, Inc.
7375 Bush Lake Rd.
Minneapolis, MN 35439
(800) 328-6366
MODEL NAME: Phox

Phillips Hearing Instrument Co.
91 McKee Dr.
Mahwah, NJ 07430
(800) 544-1677
MODEL NAME: Galaxy 3

Resound Corp.
220 Saginaw Dr.
Seaport Centre
Redwood City, CA 94063
(800) 582-HEAR
MODEL NAME: Resound

Rexton, Inc.
2415 Xenium
Plymouth, MN
(800) 876-1141
MODEL NAME: ProSys 2034

Siemens Hearing Instruments
10 Constitution Ave.
Piscataway, NJ 08854
(800) 766-4500
MODEL NAME: Triton 3000

Starkey Laboratories, Inc.
6700 Washington Ave. S.
Eden Prairie, MN 55344
(800) 328-8602
MODEL NAME: Trilogy intra

3M Corp.
3M Center—Bldg. 270-4S-16
St. Paul, MN 55144
(800) 882-3M3M
MODEL NAME: Memory Mate

Unitron Industries, Inc.
3555 Walnut St., P.O. Box 5010
Port Huron, MI 48061-5010
(800) 521-5400
MODEL NAME: Sigma System

Widex Hearing Aid Co., Inc.
35–53 24th St.
Long Island City, NY 11106
(800) 221-0188
MODEL NAME: Quattro System

environment to another, the extra investment in the new technology may be worth it. These digital aids seem to be most helpful to those who couldn't use conventional aids, who live or work in noisy settings, or who are particularly sensitive to loud sounds.

If $2,000 seems like a lot to pay for a hearing aid, you can also buy a less complex (and cheaper) version that selectively amplifies sounds by frequency while using sophisticated amplifiers to provide clear sound with low distortion. Among these options is the popular K-Amp, which is used in more than twenty brands of hearing aids. Although these aids can't be individually programmed the way a digital aid can, they can still selectively boost the amplification of quiet and high-frequency sounds. If you have only a mild hearing loss, you might find you hear well with this type of hearing aid. Those with more severe hearing loss may find that the K-Amp doesn't provide enough of a boost to the low-frequency sounds.

Keep in mind, however, that while less expensive than their digital cousins, the K-Amp versions are still not cheap. They can cost $200 more than a conventional hearing aid.

In-the-Ear Aids

This type of hearing aid is a lightweight device whose custom-made housing containing all the components fits inside the ear canal with no visible wires or tubes. It's possible to control tone but not volume with these aids, which makes them generally helpful for only mild losses.

More than half of all the hearing aids sold today are in-the-ear aids. This type of aid comes in two styles—a full-size and a half-size (called *full concha* and *half-concha*); the smaller aids tend to be more expensive, and they are harder to insert and adjust.

The good thing about an in-the-ear aid is that it won't bump into your glasses, and it can provide more power for the higher frequencies. In addition, many people find these aids are easier to put on and take off than the behind-the-ear style.

However, because they are custom-fitted to your ear, you can't try on these types of aids before you order them. Some people find the aid is uncomfortable in hot weather, and others believe they tend to break down more often than behind-the-ear styles.

HEARING AID ADD-ONS

Option	Cost	Description
Automatic gain	$100–150	Helps control distortion and interference from background noise while restraining loud sounds
Automatic signal processing	50–80	Helps reduce background noise by amplifying high-frequency conversation more than low-frequency noise
Compression	40–50	Keeps loud sounds from behind over-amplified
K-Amp	100–200	Amplifies soft to medium sounds without over-amplifying loud sounds
Pot/Trimmer	25	Allows dispenser to vary how the aid responds to various sounds
Remote control	450–900	Digital aid device that allows switching between preprogrammed settings for different listening situations (often included in package price)

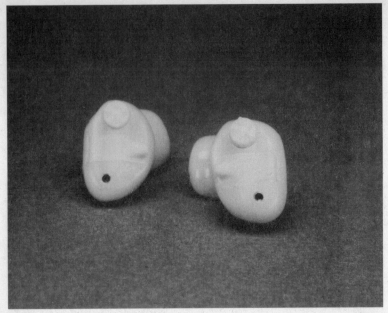

The canal aid is slightly larger than the completely in-the-canal (CIC), with volume control reachable by the wearer. (Courtesy Dahlberg, Inc.)

In-the-Canal Aids

Also called simply a *canal aid,* this device is rapidly gaining in popularity, since it fits far into the ear canal with only a small bit extending into the external ear. This is the type of hearing aid that President Ronald Reagan made popular during the 1980s. The size of the aid that protrudes into the external ear depends on the size of your ear canal.

Of these canal aids, the most recent is the completely in-the-canal aid (the peritympanic), which fits down next to the eardrum out of sight and is removed via a small transparent wire. These newest aids are extremely expensive, but they are invisible and offer acoustic and maintenance advantages.

Many people like the in-the-canal aids because they are almost invisible and more closely mimic natural sound, thanks to the position of the microphone. This microphone position also cuts down on wind noise. However, the small size also makes them harder to handle, and their battery is particularly tiny and difficult to insert. In addition, if you want to adjust the volume, you must stick your finger down into your ear and adjust the control by touch alone. It can be more difficult to fit correctly and usually requires several return visits to the dealer/dispenser. Since the smaller the aid, the higher the cost, you can imagine that this version is very expensive indeed.

You should also keep in mind that this very tiny aid does not have as much power as other, larger aids and cannot be used to correct severe hearing loss. Moreover, its small-sized battery means that you'll have to change the battery more

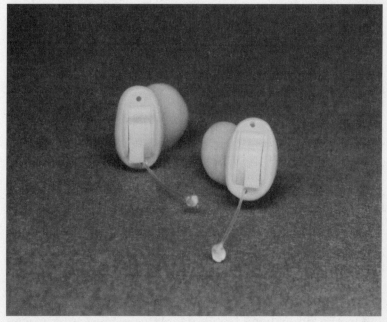

Completely in-the-ear aids are the smallest hearing aids on the market. They fit within the canal, are not visible from the outside of the ear, and are so far inside that exterior volume adjustment (i.e., without a remote control) is not possible. (Courtesy Dalhberg, Inc.)

often. And although larger aids can make room for a tele-phone coil to pick up the electric signals over the phone, the in-the-canal aid is too small to pack in such extras.

Behind-the-Ear Aids

Less popular are the behind-the-ear aids that include a microphone, amplifier, and receiver inside a small curved case worn behind the ear that's connected to the earmold by a short plastic tube. The earmold extends into the ear canal from a quarter to three quarters of an inch. Some models have both tone and volume control plus a telephone pickup device.

Though they account for only about 20 percent of the market (many people view them as unattractive and out-of-date), they do offer a few advantages.

- This style doesn't require as much maintenance, since the earmolds can handle everyday trauma better than smaller, more delicate models.
- It is easily interchangeable if you have to take one in for servicing.
- It is more powerful, and therefore more effective, for those whose hearing loss ranges from mild to severe.
- It is easier to handle than the smaller aids.
- It has longer-lasting batteries that need to be changed only once a month.
- It can provide better sound quality because it has room for more circuitry.
- It tends to be more reliable, since it doesn't come in con-tact with ear wax.

On the other hand, some people who must wear glasses find that the aids interfere with their fit, pushing against the glasses. Others don't have enough space behind their ears for such a device to fit comfortably. And while the microphone's position outside the ear minimizes feedback, it can pick up and amplify the sound of wind.

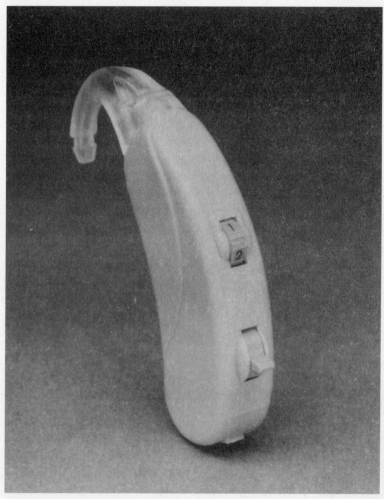

The "behind the ear" hearing aid, as the name implies, is worn behind the ear. It can produce more volume for those with more severe hearing loss. (Courtesy Dahlberg, Inc.)

Eyeglass Models

This model is much the same as the behind-the-ear aid, except that the case fits into an eyeglass frame instead of resting behind the ear. Although this means that the eyeglass frame needs to be slightly larger, modern miniaturized parts result in an eyeglass frame that is not too obtrusive. Still, not very many people choose to buy this type of aid.

Those who do favor this type believe that the aid is less conspicuous than other models, although there is a tube that travels from the temple of the glasses to the earmold. Bone-conduction hearing aids are also available in the eyeglass model.

Still, it can be difficult to fit this type of hearing aid. You must purchase a new set of eyeglass frames (and sometimes lenses) and then work with both the hearing aid dispenser and your optician to get the devices properly adjusted.

Because eyeglass models tend to need more repairs than other models, you'll find it quite annoying because when either the eyeglasses or the aid needs repair, you'll have to have a backup extra set of glasses and hearing aids. And you might find the eye-and-ears connection annoying for those times when you might want to wear glasses without fussing with a hearing aid.

CROS or Crossover System

This type of hearing aid system is often used in conjunction with the eyeglass model discussed above. The CROS (contralateral routing of signal) system features a microphone behind the impaired ear that feeds the amplified signal to the better ear, eliminating "head shadow" (which occurs when the head blocks sound from the better ear). This system may help make speech easier to understand for those with a high-frequency loss in both ears.

Bi-CROS systems use two microphones (one above each ear) that send signals to a single amplifier. Sound then travels to a single receiver, which transfers it to the better ear via a conventional earmold.

On-the-Body Aids

These hearing aids feature a larger microphone, amplifier, and power supply inside a case carried inside a pocket or attached to clothing. The external receiver attaches directly to the earmold; its power comes through a flexible wire from the amplifier. Although larger than other aids, on-the-body hearing aids are also more powerful and easier to adjust than smaller devices. They are not very popular, but some are still used today for people with profound hearing loss and for very young children.

If you are almost totally deaf, you'll find that you need the extra boost in power available only from a body aid. Further, anyone who has any type of physical disability that interferes with the ability to handle tiny parts can benefit from a body aid. On the other hand, such a large aid is bulky and visible. It is rarely used for cases of age-related hearing loss.

Monaural/Binaural Aids

Monaural hearing aids include any aid that provides sound to just one ear, whereas binaural aids include two complete hearing devices, one in each ear. Some wearers find that the binaural system increases direction sense and helps separate sound from unwanted background noise. On the other hand, recent research suggests that going binaural may not be the best choice for everyone.

You may have a hearing loss in both ears, but one ear still hears better; if this is the case, you may have adapted over the years so that you understand speech by relying more heavily on the better ear. Wearing hearing aids to amplify speech on both the good and poor ears may interfere with your comprehension. Still, most people with hearing loss in both ears will need two hearing aids, especially in noisy environments.

NEW TECHNOLOGY: MAGNETIC AIDS

The next generation of hearing aids may eliminate the amplifier and speaker in favor of a tiny magnet mounted on a silicone disk similar to a contact lens, which will rest right on the eardrum. Called the Earlens, it is designed to be held in place by a thin film of oil. Users will wear a wireless microphone either in the ear or on a necklace that will pick up sounds and convert them into magnetic signals, making the magnet vibrate. As the Earlens vibrates, so will the eardrum, transmitting normal-sounding tones to the middle and inner ears.

Other researchers are bypassing the middle ear entirely by surgically implanting a tiny magnet in the inner ear. Normally when we hear, the sound vibrates the eardrum, which vibrates the bones of the middle ear, traveling through the oval window into the cochlea of the inner ear. Researchers attach a magnet to the round window, opening a second pathway to the inner ear. An electromagnetic coil implanted in bone behind the ear would vibrate the implanted magnet. Unlike the Earlens, this magnetic implant would not block the normal hearing pathway.

CARING FOR YOUR HEARING AID

A hearing aid is a delicate, high-tech electronic device. It should last about five years, with gentle handling, occasional preventive maintenance, and a few simple precautions. By taking care of the aid, you can lower your maintenance and repair costs considerably. Here are a few general suggestions for the proper care of your hearing aid:

- Heat and cold can damage a hearing aid. Don't wear it under a hair dryer or store it near a heat source, and keep it off windowsills where it can be exposed to sunlight. Don't wear it for more than a few minutes in very cold weather.

- Avoid wearing the aid in the rain or when sweating a great deal, although drops of rain aren't as harmful as mist and vapor—so keep it out of steamy bathrooms and kitchens. Don't inadvertently spray it with hair spray. *Never wear the aid while bathing.*
- Turn the aid off every time you remove it.
- Keep the aid in a plastic bag with a silica gel overnight, to help absorb moisture.
- Turn the aid off and remove the battery when you're not using it. Remove dead batteries immediately.
- Don't handle the hearing aid roughly, and try to avoid knocking it onto the floor.
- Wash the earmold with soapy water occasionally, but never immerse the mechanical parts of the hearing aid.
- Never use alcohol or cleaning fluid to clean the earmold or instrument.
- Protect it from dust, since small particles can clog up the microphone openings.
- Watch out for wax build-up in the small holes of the earmold. If you produce lots of wax, ask your dispenser about a wax guard, a small screen that can catch wax before it becomes wedged in the hearing aid.
- Clean the battery compartment and connections with a pencil eraser.
- Replace the tubing on behind-the-ear aids when it becomes yellowed or brittle.
- Replace cracked wiring on body hearing aids right away.
- Keep spare batteries with you, and store extras in a cool, dry place.
- Insert only dry, room-temperature batteries in the aid.
- Don't keep more than a month's supply of batteries at one time.
- Take your hearing aid to your dealer/dispenser for a check-up and cleaning once a year.

TIPS ON CONSERVING HEARING AID BATTERIES

- Allow your batteries to dry out overnight by opening the battery compartment of the hearing aid.
- Don't carry batteries in the same pocket as loose change; the coins will drain the batteries.
- Keep extra batteries on hand and change them as soon as you notice the sound getting weaker or distorted.
- Dispose of batteries carefully so pets and children don't swallow them.

Hearing Aid Features

You may be interested in investigating some extra hearing aid features, such as telecoil circuitry and tone control, which can be used with certain "assistive listening systems and devices" (see Chapter 8).

The telecoil (or T-coil) is a tiny electrical component that can sense magnetic forces generated by another coil nearby, such as the speaker coil in a telephone or a loop or wire around the room or around a person's neck. The telecoil was developed for use with the telephone to allow clearer sound reception for hard-of-hearing consumers.

When you flip the T-switch on your hearing aid, you disconnect the aid's microphone. This allows the aid to receive magnetic signals directly from the telephone, transmitting them to the amplifier. This helps shut out background noise and eliminates the feedback that is common when using the telephone with a conventional hearing aid.

T-switches also have become important with the advent of assistive listening devices and assistive listening systems (see Chapter 7). More and more, public areas (such as churches, theaters, meeting rooms, and so forth) have been fitted with assistive listening systems to help people with hearing problems. When such a system is in place, the hearing aid wearer can turn on the T-mode to receive sound directly from the listening system in the room. Or, where certain public places feature FM or infrared systems, the wearer may use a special receiver to connect with the hearing aid in the T-mode. In much the same way, assistive listening devices use the T-switch to improve hearing of TV and radio.

Not all hearing aids have a telecoil (most canal or in-the-ear aids do not). However, most behind-the-ear and all body aids have telecoils. Because there are no regulations or standards regarding telecoils, they can vary as much as 30 dB in maximum sound output.

Compression circuits

If you've ever had problems with a hearing aid in a crowded environment, this could be for you. These circuits can provide easier listening in the presence of noise for almost anyone by cutting their power when your surroundings get loud.

Noise-reduction circuits

Also called *automatic signal processing*, these circuits can sense rising noise levels and automatically adjust themselves to reduce the effects of these sounds. The more sophisticated the circuit, the more expensive.

High-frequency aids

This model extends into the high pitches for much clearer speech comprehension and easier listening to music and noise.

Implantable aids

Unlike the cochlear implant, which we will discuss at the end of this chapter, the implantable aids are surgically implanted within the ear canal in the hope of overcoming many of the drawbacks of conventional in-the-ear hearing aids. (These aids have a tendency toward acoustic feedback and discomfort.) The implantable aid effectively removes this feedback problem by eliminating acoustic coupling, and should provide greater comfort. They can be more acceptable to those who need amplification but cannot (or choose not) to use currently available hearing aids.

Problems with Hearing Aids

For those who do get an aid, too many end up not wearing it. Many people wrongly assume that a hearing aid will solve their hearing problems. When they realize that using an aid isn't simply a matter of popping one in the ear, the aid is often abandoned. The key to success with a hearing aid is lots of practice coupled with hearing therapy, counseling, and a positive attitude.

Painful aids

Many people with hearing problems say everything seems loud after they receive a hearing aid, but this is because they have lived for so long with a hearing deficit they have forgotten how loud "normal" sound can be. If you have worn your hearing aid for several weeks and you experience pain or discomfort, you should return to your dealer/dispenser for a readjustment.

You may notice that your earmold feels a bit uncomfortable at first, which is normal. However, if there is redness, irritation, soreness, or swelling, you should go back to the dealer and have the earmold adjusted.

Excess wax

Many people complain that they have much more ear wax after they get a hearing aid. It is true that wearing an earmold seems to boost the production of ear wax. Actually, people who don't wear hearing aids have wax that falls out of their ears naturally. When you wear an earmold, the wax can't fall out on its own, and you actually retain ear wax. You may need to visit a doctor to have this excess wax removed.

If you have a problem with your aid

Your hearing aid is as delicate in its own way as the human hearing mechanism. Even with excellent care, most aids last only about five years, because the many tiny components can break. For example, if your aid sounds weak and scratchy, or it whistles, buzzes, or clicks off and on, this is *not* simply typical hearing aid behavior that you just have to learn to live with.

If you're having a problem with your aid and you can't fix it yourself—and you should never try to open the hearing aid case—then you must return it to the hearing aid dealer or dispensing audiologist. Although these experts can fix many problems in the office, sometimes the aids must be sent back to the factory for several weeks. If necessary, you can borrow an aid from the dealer.

Cochlear Implants

Four-year-old Amy stands in front of her mirror, smiling at her reflection in ballet slippers and tutu. As she listens to the music in her mind, she envisions herself up on stage, dancing the lead to the *Nutcracker Suite*.

A year ago, Amy lost her hearing after a serious ear infection. Her parents had feared that she would never reach her dream of dancing the ballet. Today, with the aid of a special electronic device called a cochlear implant, her dream is much closer to coming true.

Amy is one of a growing number of children in this country who have been given a cochlear implant, a new surgical treatment for hearing loss. Unlike a hearing aid, which simply amplifies sound, an implant works much like an artificial human cochlea in the inner ear, helping to send sound from the ear to the brain.

Surgically implanted in the mastoid bone, it stimulates the hearing nerve and allows a hard-of-hearing person to hear some sound. Still, *the implant does not restore normal hearing.*

For people like Amy, the implant does offer the means of hearing speech and sounds—something that no other type of hearing aid can do. However, the use of cochlear implants, especially for children, remains controversial. Members of the deaf community and hearing specialists debate whether the benefits outweigh the risks and limitations of these devices. Because the device is implanted during surgery, it subjects young children to the typical risks of general anesthesia. What's more, no one can estimate how well any particular individual will hear with the implant.

The deaf community is also concerned about possible emotional and psychological problems. After receiving the implant, some people say they feel isolated—alienated from the deaf community but not truly belonging to the hearing world, either. Many deaf individuals are concerned about the message that hearing parents may inadvertently send their deaf children—that deafness is unacceptable, that only a hearing child can be loved.

On the other hand, the implant potentially has the ability to restore some hearing by bypassing the damaged hair cells and helping to establish some degree of hearing from direct stimulation of the hearing nerve, helping a deaf child to communicate better with the hearing world.

All cochlear implants have the same basic equipment. A microphone is worn behind the ear to pick up sound, routing it along a wire to a speech processor that can be worn in a small shoulder pouch, a pocket, or a belt. The processor amplifies the sound, filters out background noise, and transforms the sound into digital signals before sending it to a transmitter worn behind the ear. The impulses are then sent via electrodes inside a narrow, flexible tube that has been inserted into the cochlea. Implants may feature as many as 22 electrodes that transmit impulses to the auditory nerve and on to the brain, which then interprets the signal as individual sounds.

During the operation, the surgeon makes an incision behind the ear and opens the mastoid bone (the ridge on your skull behind the ear). The surgeon then inserts the receiver/stimulator in the mastoid bone and threads the electrodes into the cochlea.

The operation usually lasts about three hours, and the hospital stay is about a day or two. After the surgical wounds have healed, patients return to the implant clinic to be fitted with the external parts of the implant—the speech processor, microphone, and transmitter. A clinician tunes the speech processor, setting levels of stimulation for each electrode (from soft to loud).

Then you begin an important training period, learning how to interpret the sounds that you hear through the implant. Training may take only months, or it might take years, depending on how well you can interpret the sounds.

Still, the implant is not for everyone. Before you can be eligible for a device, you must be evaluated by specialists at an implant clinic. The experts will give you extensive hearing tests to figure out how well you hear with an aid. The Food and Drug Administration (FDA), which regulates the implants, has limited it to people with severe to profound hearing loss. They have set this limit because the implants cost so much (a minimum of $25,000), and their effectiveness cannot be predicted on an individual basis.

If powerful hearing aids can't improve your hearing, a physician performs a physical exam and takes a CT scan to evaluate whether your inner ear is suitable for an implant. If your cochlea has been scarred by injury or disease, you won't benefit very much from an implant. Specialists also check for signs of an ear infection, and assess whether or not you can withstand general anesthesia. Some physicians may order psychological evaluations to determine if your expectations are unrealistic. Experts look for patients who are highly motivated and yet who understand what the implant might and might not be able to do. If you pass all these evaluations, you're ready for an implant.

FDA REQUIREMENTS FOR COCHLEAR IMPLANTS

The FDA regulates medical devices to ensure their safety and effectiveness, and has set a number of requirements for anyone considering a cochlear implant. They require that implant candidates must:

- Be severely to profoundly deaf
- Experience no significant benefit from hearing aids
- Be at least two years old (the age when specialists can verify the severity of a child's deafness)

In addition, candidates should:
- Be strong enough to withstand general anesthesia
- Be highly motivated and realistic about benefits
- Have an unscarred cochlea
- Have no current ear infection

Because the device has a limited number of electrodes, it cannot hope to match the complexity of a person's 15,000 hair cells. As a result, sounds heard through an implant have been described as "robot-like" or "cartoon-like." Still, these implants have significantly improved the communication skills of many deafened adults.

Most profoundly deaf patients who receive an implant can hear medium and loud sounds, including speech, at comfortable listening levels. Many can communicate by combining the sound clues from the implant with speechreading and watching for facial cues. According to studies by the FDA, almost all adults improve their communication skills if they combine speechreading and implant use, and some can understand spoken words without speechreading.

More than half the adult recipients who lost their hearing after they learned to speak can understand some speech without speechreading after a cochlear implant, according to Noel Cohen, an ear, nose, and throat specialist at New York University. About 30 percent can understand spoken words well enough to use the telephone.

Those who experience the most difficulty in learning to use the implant are children who were born deaf or who lost their hearing before acquiring speech. However, recent research suggests that most of these children are still able to learn spoken language and understand speech using the implant. Many are able to attend regular schools rather than schools for deaf children.

The implants have proven effective in improving deaf people's ability to speak intelligibly, understand other people's words, and read lips, according to researchers at the University of California at San Diego and San Diego State University. For three years scientists studied patients between the ages of 18 and 60 who had recently received cochlear implants. During this time patients showed increased confidence to take jobs or go to school in preparation for work, and they also experienced a steady upward growth in personal income.

In clinical studies with children over age two, those implanted with the device detected medium-to-loud conversation and environmental sounds (such as doorbells or car horns). Many were better able to identify the timing and rhythm of speech. A few recognized speech without speechreading, and others found the implant made it easier to speechread. Training and experience with the device often improved the child's own speech.

Of the 200 children in the study, 33 had at least one reaction or complication—mostly transient loud noises (15), skin irritation (5), ear infection (5), and problems related to surgery (5).

Many factors influence how well a person responds to a cochlear implant. In general, the later in life you lose your hearing and the shorter the duration of that loss, the more speech you are likely to understand with an implant. If your auditory nerve is healthy, you also are more likely to understand sounds with an implant. Good postoperative training can make a great deal of difference in how well you can understand sounds.

FOR MORE INFORMATION

The National Hearing Aid Society operates a helpline for anyone who needs information about hearing loss and hearing aids. You can call to find qualified, competent hearing aid specialists or to ask questions about hearing devices, dispensing, and service. They'll send you a consumer information kit, which includes a regional edition of the membership directory of the Hearing Aid Society, plus a booklet covering such topics as how hearing works, signs of hearing loss, and types of hearing aids. The group also offers information on assistive listening devices, requirements for entering the hearing aid profession, statistics on hearing loss and hearing instruments, and so on. The helpline does not provide medical advice, recommend specific products, or quote prices. Although financial assistance is not available through the helpline, staffers can provide a list of possible financial resources. All services and materials provided are free. Callers may use the helpline numbers (1-800-521-5247; in Michigan, 1-313-478-2610 Monday through Friday, 9 A.M. to 4:30 P.M. EST).

7

Other Assistive Devices

If you have any sort of hearing loss, chances are you are well aware of the particular instances when it's especially hard for you to comprehend conversation or important sounds. Fortunately, in our technological society there are different kinds of devices that can be used to help you hear better. Hearing aids are only one of them.

Today you can take advantage of a variety of assistive listening systems, devices, communication aids, and alerting devices. You can even obtain a "hearing ear" dog trained to react to sound. The dogs are trained to be sensitive to certain noises and to run back and forth between the source of the noise and the master.

Alerting Devices

If you retain some ability to hear sounds, you might not need anything fancier than a wind-up alarm clock, for instance, since these often generate plenty of noise and are louder than a buzzer on most electric clocks. Alternatively, you could try using a timer set to turn on lights at a certain time. If everyday devices around the house aren't practical in your case, you may be interested in some form of special alerting device.

Visual Alarms

Some of the most common assistive products are the alerting devices that warn of particular sounds (such as a doorbell, crying baby, telephone, timer) by activating a visual light signal. The visual alarms often feature one or more flashing lights (one lamp or all the lights in the house). The lights are turned on either through direct wiring or by using a signal transmitted through the building's wiring system. Some systems can even alert you to different sounds by using different light patterns for each sound.

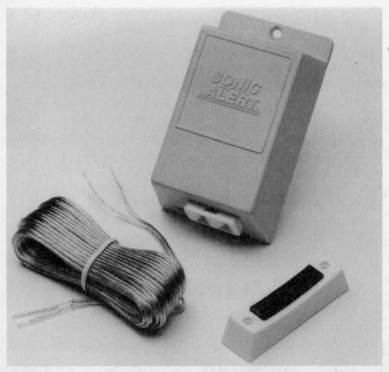

Doorbell ringers coordinate with house lights to announce a visitor at the door for people with hearing problems. (Courtesy Sonic Alert)

Audio alarms, such as ordinary clock radios or electronic alarms, have also been adapted to flash one or several lights. Lights can be set to go off when someone knocks at the door. Very bright strobe lights can be set to alert you when the telephone rings or when a smoke alarm goes off. And if you are driving in your car, you can buy a small device to alert you that your turn signal has been left on, since the standard alerting sound can be very hard to hear.

Vibrator Alarms

Sometimes vibrators are used as alarms. An alarm clock is connected to a vibrator under the mattress or pillow; it replaces the normal alarm buzzer on the clock. Your doorbell can also be hooked into this vibrating system. Other devices vibrate a wristband when the phone rings or in the presence of certain other sounds.

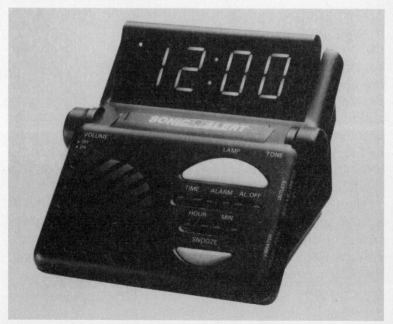

The "Sonic Boom" vibrating alarm can alert a person with hearing problems by vibrating the person's bed. (Siemens Hearing Instruments, Inc.)

Telephone Ring Alternatives

If you have trouble hearing the phone ring when you're in another part of the house and you don't want an alerting device to turn on your lights, make sure that your ringing device on the phone is turned up to full volume. (You'll find the adjustment knob or wheel underneath the phone, or on the side of a wall model.)

You can have the telephone company install a louder ringing device in your phone or get a ring at a lower pitch. You can also have the phone company install extra ringing devices in other parts of your house, or simply add another phone.

Assistive Listening Systems

Even with the most powerful hearing aid, if you have a hearing problem you'll probably have a fair amount of trouble hearing in a large chamber such as an auditorium. Background noise and vibration can compound your hearing loss and interfere with your ability to pick up specific sounds. Because of this, large public meeting rooms, concert halls, auditoriums, and churches are sometimes equipped with one of a number of different alternative listening-device systems, including induction systems, infrared systems, audio loop systems, direct audio input (DAI), and extension microphones (including AM and FM transmission systems).

Many public places advertise this service; all you have to do is to ask which section of the room you should sit. If you don't have a hearing aid with a T-switch to take advantage of these systems, you may be able to borrow a receiver that has been specially equipped.

Induction

It's possible to generate a magnetic field capable of transmitting sound from a coil connected to a sound source that transmits the sound to a specially equipped hearing aid. This coil can be a loop of wire strung around a room, worn around the neck, embedded in a small, flat plastic device hooked over the ear, or placed in the receiver of a compatible telephone. A second coil that picks up this magnetic signal is built into many hearing aids. Called a telecoil, it is activated by using the T-switch on hearing aids.

One advantage of the T-switch capability is that the microphone in the hearing aid is usually turned off, so background noise doesn't interfere with the sound from the induction system. For hearing aids without a T-switch, special receivers are available that have a telecoil that picks up and amplifies sound.

An induction-loop *system* refers to a loop of wire placed around an entire room that is connected to a microphone and an amplifier. The system's microphone picks up sound and changes it into electrical energy that is then amplified and sent through the coil of a wire (or induction loop) strung around the room. The electrical energy flowing through the wire coil creates a magnetic field that can be picked up by the T-coil of a hearing aid.

Direct Audio Input (DAI)

Direct audio input makes it possible to transfer sound directly to the hearing aid, taking advantage of the aid's amplification and eliminating through-the-air noise. With some aids the DAI signal can be heard while in the T-mode; turning off the microphone can further eliminate background noise. The hearing aid must be equipped to accept a DAI attachment.

Extension Microphones

This type of assistive device extends the microphone closer to the sound source rather than having you rely solely on the microphone built into your hearing aid. Because microphone sensitivity drops rapidly with distance, an extension makes the signal stronger and tends to minimize background noise. There are several types of extension microphones: hard-wired, amplified, and wireless.

Hard-wired microphones consist solely of an additional microphone connected via cable and coupled to a hearing aid either by earphones, induction device (neck loop or ear hook), or DAI. Most devices need an amplifier worn in your pocket, on your belt, or in your hand, although palm-sized models combine the microphone with the amplifier. Super-directional models are also available that allow you to pick up a voice six to ten feet away if there isn't too much background noise.

For those who need less amplification and who don't wear a hearing aid, you can use an *amplified* microphone attached to a battery-powered pocket or belt amplifier. The amplifier can be connected to the ear by an earphone or a built-in speaker held close to the ear. As with hard-wired micro-phones, the amplified microphone cable can be as long as you need.

The *wireless* (personal FM system) is considered to be the ultimate in extension microphones. This transmitter can broadcast 150 to 300 feet without connecting cables. The transmitter can be connected directly to the source of the sound, such as a TV set or a microphone; the sound is carried on a specific FM radio frequency through the air until it reaches an FM receiver tuned to the same fre-quency. (The FCC has set aside the FM frequencies between 72 and 76 megahertz for such use by both public and private systems.)

When the FM signal reaches the receiver, it's changed into electrical energy, which can be picked up by a person wearing either a headset or a hearing aid. If your aid has a telecoil, it can connect to a necklace loop attached to the receiver. Alter-natively, if your hearing aid has DAI capability, it can be linked to the FM systems with a special attachment called a boot, which fits on the bottom of a behind-the-ear aid and connects to the receiver by a wire.

With characteristically good sound quality, the FM system can be very helpful for those with severe or profound hearing problems, and can provide for another microphone in addition to the built-in device.

A similar system uses an AM signal so that you could listen to an AM receiver headset or a portable radio to sounds transmitted on an AM radio. The AM transmitter can also be connected to a public address system. Unfortunately, this system is open to the same interference that disrupts regular AM radio broadcasts.

Infrared Systems

Some large rooms and public places are equipped with a P.A. system that is plugged into an infrared light emitter that transmits sound via invisible light waves. An infrared transmitter can be connected directly to a sound source or a microphone; the transmitter then uses harmless infrared light rays to transmit sound to portable infrared receivers (available with headphones or "stethoscopes" that then change the signal into electrical energy and back into sound.

If you don't have a severe hearing loss, you may use the headphones without a hearing aid. But if the loss is more serious, you may want to connect a hearing aid directly to an infrared receiver or use the aid's telecoil capability together with a neck loop.

With a neck loop, the infrared receiver sends an electrical signal to the loop, where it creates an electromagnetic signal picked up by the hearing aid. This signal is converted into electrical energy and then converted into sound at the aid's receiver.

Unlike FM transmission, light waves do not pass through walls and are not affected by neighboring radio frequency

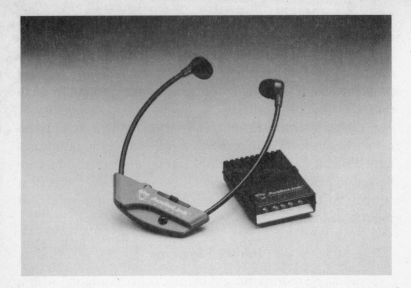

An infrared listening system such as this one transmits auditory signals to the hard-of-hearing listener via radio frequencies, over either a speaker or a headset as a way of enhancing TV or stereo sound. The headset can also be used in compatible public facilities. (Courtesy Siemens Hearing Instruments, Inc.)

signals. However, infrared transmission may be affected by intense sunlight. Infrared devices are most helpful if you have a mild to moderately severe hearing loss.

Telephone Aids

The telephone is often one of the biggest communication obstacles for those who have hearing problems, since the sound is often distorted and visual cues are nonexistent. One way around this is to use a fax machine whenever possible. Computer e-mail communication systems also can be a handy choice for many people with hearing problems.

Of course, sometimes you almost *have* to use a telephone.

In these cases it may help to have a hearing aid with telecoil capability. The hearing aid telecoil was developed in America to take advantage of a defect in the telephone's design—the fact that the magnetic signal leaks. That leak can be picked up by a hearing aid equipped with a telecoil. Simply flip your hearing aid's T-switch to shut off its microphone; the telecoil then picks up the magnetic signal from the phone and transfers it to the amplifier, eliminating the feedback and background noise.

Unfortunately, some older telephones don't work well with a T-switch because when they were built, they were "shielded" as a way of preventing wiretapping. If your phone has been manufactured since 1989, however, it will be compatible to a T-switch. In the United States all new models of home telephones and all public phones must be compatible to telecoil circuitry. By law as of May 1, 1994, all phones in all workplaces must be hearing-aid compatible (HAC), in addition to all "essential" phones (such as coin-operated phones and those designated for emergency use). Retrofitting a phone to make it hearing-aid compatible costs about $40.

It's important to realize that some telephones have better telecoil capability than others; make sure you have the opportunity to return a phone that doesn't work well with your hearing aid.

Portable Adapters

Another type of telephone device slips over the receiver and converts the audio signal into a strong magnetic signal that is then picked up by the T-coil of a hearing aid. There is also an attachable amplifier that combines both types.

Still, reception from a T-switch–equipped hearing aid is not perfect, since there is usually some distortion. Unlike assistive-device systems used in auditoriums and other public places, the telephone was not built specifically for this type of transmission. Moreover, the quality of the T-circuit varies widely among different brands of hearing aids.

Telephone Amplifiers

If you run into too much trouble with your telecoil, you can always attach an amplifier to your telephone so you don't need to use your aid. You can buy an *amplifying handset* with an amplifier built into the telephone receiver that boosts the volume without distorting sound. It will have an adjustment wheel to increase sound as necessary. Some models have another push button that boosts volume. There is also a modular portable amplified handset that may be substituted for unamplified handsets of similar modular units when you're traveling.

The disadvantage of this type of assistive device is that you'll need to remove your hearing aid, unless you are wearing an in-the-air aid that is placed deeply enough to allow a tight seal between your ear and the phone. Even then you may hear the squeal of hearing aid feedback.

If portability is important, there are several options from which you can choose. One type of *attachable portable amplifier* slips over the handset receiver and increases the audio signal; the small box-shaped model plugs into a modular fitting at the base of the phone and amplifies the signal there. However, some say the quality is not quite as good as a built-in amplifier.

If you wear a hearing aid when you're on the phone, you might run into feedback, an unpleasant squealing sound. There are telephone attachments that minimize the feedback that occurs when the receiver is held against a hearing aid. Less expensive approaches include a plastic foam-filled cap designed for telephone comfort that can be slipped over the receiver.

For many people, these devices have proven invaluable. "I have a mild hearing loss in one ear from standing next to a big gun during the Korean War," explains James, 61. "I get by without hearing aids by paying attention and reading lips, but I have more trouble when using the phone. By purchasing a simple telephone amplifier from Radio Shack, I can adjust it to pick up the softest whisper all the way when talking to my son, who speaks so loud I can hear him even without a telephone."

FOR MORE INFORMATION

For more information about hearing aids and telephones, contact the Tele-Consumer Hotline, a nonprofit, independent, and impartial telephone consumer-information service that provides free telephone assistance and publications on special telephone equipment, TDD (telecommunications device for the deaf) directories, and TDD/voice relay services. Contact: Tele-Consumer Hotline, 1910 K. St. NW, Suite 610, Washington, DC 20006 or call (202) 223-4371 (voice/TDD) or (800) 332-1244.

Television Devices

Listening to TV can be frustrating if you have a hearing loss. Even if you hear well enough to make out most of what is going on, straining to hear can be exhausting. There are several devices that have been developed to boost your ability to hear. Unlike a standard earphone on a TV, some of these devices don't eliminate the TV's speaker, and people without a hearing problem can watch the same program.

If your TV set is *hard-wired*, you can simply plug the accompanying earphones into the listening jack on the television. Alternatively, a cable can be connected from the listening jack of the TV to the microphone jack of a portable amplifier. If there is no listening jack on the TV, an extension microphone can be mounted near the TV speaker.

A small portable radio called a *TV band radio* that receives both UHF and VHF audio broadcasts of the TV usually has better sound quality. You can simply place the radio near your chair as you watch, and use either the radio's speaker or its earphone.

If your hearing aid is equipped with a T-switch, you can use an *audio induction loop* in conjunction with your TV. The amplifier converts the TV audio signal to an induction signal, and transmits it to either a neck-loop or a loop system around the wall or under your chair. Loop and/or wire can be permanently installed, which avoids a cable stretching across the room.

Finally, you can borrow the *infrared* technology used for TV remote-control units with a device that utilizes a microphone to transform the TV sound into infrared light, transmitting it to a stethoscope or clip-on receiver; sound is transmitted to the ear via an earphone, neck loop, or DAI. While you use this, it blocks noise around you and improves listening ability.

Alternatively, you may want to invest in a *telecaption decoder* for your TV (or buy a TV with a built-in decoder). These devices attach to your TV set and interpret "closed caption" signals that are broadcast at the same time as the TV program, converting them to subtitles across the bottom of your TV screen. You'll find these subtitles on all major TV station networks, as well as some independent stations, cable TV, and Canadian broadcasters. Because viewers who don't have hearing problems might find ordinary subtitles (open captions) distracting, you'll need a special telecaption decoder to see the closed captions on your screen.

Manufactured and distributed by the National Captioning Institute, the devices are compatible with all TVs, videocassette recorders, and cable hookups. They can be turned off to view programs without subtitles if you wish. Since 1980 NCI has developed several generations of decoders, and together with ITT Corp., they have developed an integrated circuit chip that allows TV manufacturers to provide built-in

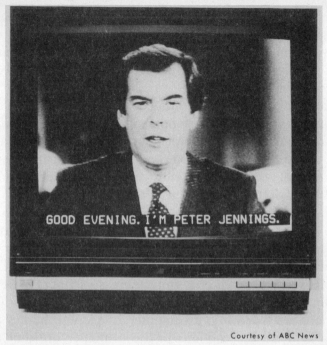

Courtesy of ABC News

Closed captions for captioned television programs appear as written dialogue at the bottom of the TV screen. (Courtesy National Captioning Institute, Inc.)

decoding capability. Soon decoders will be obsolete because a new federal law requires that TV sets bigger than 13 inches have a built-in system.

Captioning

Closed captioning was introduced in 1980 and is now used in more than 70 percent of prime-time programming on networks and cable TV in addition to local and national news, sports, and political events. A large number of videos are also now available in closed-captioned versions.

A free service of TV and cable networks and home video producers, captioning is funded by corporations, foundations, the government, producers, networks, and program sponsors. In addition, people interested in closed-captioned programs may join NCI's Caption Club, whose membership dues are used to fund captioning of TV programs that reflect viewers' preferences.

Captioning was at first limited to previously taped programs, but in 1984 the development of computer technology had reached the point that real-time captioning became available for live broadcasts. Most captioning is done at the headquarters of the NCI in Falls Church, Virginia, and at WGBH-TV in Boston. When captioning prerecorded programs, an editor records captions on a magnetic disk that is then sent to the TV broadcaster, where it is inserted into the TV signal. It takes about 30 hours to caption a one-hour program and costs about $2,500.

For live TV programs for which there is a script prepared in advance, captions are prepared before the program airs. The captions are typed into a computer, and when the live program is aired, the captions in the computer are sent to a machine that adds them to the TV signal.

For live programs without prepared scripts (such as debates and news conferences), it's possible to create captions as the program is being aired. A court stenographer enters phonetic symbols into a computer that then translates the symbols into words and beams them through the network to viewers about four seconds after words are spoken. Although this system works fairly well, captions cannot be edited and mistakes occasionally appear.

Published TV schedules usually mark captioned programs with a C or CC; the TeleCaption decoder itself provides a Program Listing Update Service, which is a daily listing of captioned programs and sponsors.

You can buy these decoders (which are tax-deductible) from the National Captioning Institute, various other stores and organizations (addresses at the end of this chapter), organizations for people with hearing problems, and assistive-devices centers. You may also be able to lease a decoder through your cable system operator, who may be able to offer you a cable converter/decoder.

Text-Telephones (TT)

The text-telephone (TT) or telecommunication device for the deaf (TDD) is a mechanical device that allows you to type phone messages over the telephone network. TT is a generic term for text-typewriter, which transmits typewritten messages over the telephone wires. The initials TT used to be called TDD, which replaces the still earlier term TTY, which referred specifically to teletypewriter machines. The TDD number is the same as a TT number.

A TT is basically a visual typewriter, connected to a telephone line by a modular plug or acoustic modem. The conversation is displayed on a screen moving from right to left above the keyboard. You can add a printer to provide a permanent paper record of all messages transmitted and received. Of course, with this system you can only call other people with TTs, but more and more public businesses and organizations are adding TT numbers.

The original TDD was invented in 1964 by Robert Weitbrecht, a deaf physicist and licensed ham radio operator, together with James Marsters, a deaf orthodontist. The two wanted to investigate the ways a hard-of-hearing person could communicate by using a TTY with a radio or telephone. Working together in California, the two decided a telephone system would be more logical since many hard-of-hearing people already had telephones in their homes. A radio system, they reasoned, would require a deaf person to get a license from the FCC.

In some states phone companies lend or sell TTs at subsidized prices, and more and more public agencies are installing them. In addition, relay services are available to connect TT users and voice calls through an interpreter. By law, every state must have a relay service in place.

Telephone companies usually offer reduced long-distance rates when a TT is used, since it takes longer to type than it does to talk. Some states have introduced legislation that would require free or reduced-price TTs be made available to those who need them. Otherwise, a TT may cost between $150 and $600 depending on which additional options are included, such as answering machines, printers, or call waiting.

TT and Computers

Because TTs and computers use different codes for the letters of the alphabet and other characters, they cannot normally communicate. However, you can equip your personal computer with a modem to make it function like a TT. (A modem is a device that allows a computer to use a telephone line to transmit information to other computers with compatible modems).

Most TTs with built-in modems can understand only transmissions in the Baudot code. Personal computers use the ASCII code, and modems designed for use with a computer accommodate only that code. However, there are several modems available that have the ability to communicate in both Baudot and ASCII codes.

Today there are a wide variety of other TT products. Some come in small, lightweight, portable sizes; some have built-in answering machines that respond only to TT calls. There is also an answering machine that can respond to both voice and TT calls.

In 1989, IBM introduced the Phone-Communicator, a system that allows a person with a TT to communicate over phone lines with anyone owning an IBM-compatible personal computer. The Phone Communicator includes an automatic answer mode capable of recording messages from Touch-Tone telephones and TT callers.

New devices include communication systems that use Touch-Tone phones to allow one party in the conversation to spell out messages, or voice synthesizers that allow you to type in a message and have the unit speak for you. (A few companies that offer these new products are listed at the end of this chapter.)

Of course, no matter what assistive devices you decide to try, remember that they can make your life easier, but you can't expect them to cure all of your communication problems. In the next chapter you'll find some suggestions on adapting to your hearing loss and how to make the most of your communication.

Assistive Devices

Please note that this list is as up to date as possible at the time this book was prepared. Inclusion of a particular product or service does not indicate endorsement; exclusion does not indicate a negative rating.

Information

Most of the devices discussed in this chapter are not sold in stores, except for regular burglar alarms. If your local dispenser can't help you, you can write or call for free information from the following places:

Better Hearing Institute
5021-B Blacklick Rd.
Annandale, VA 22003
(800) EAR-WELL

National Association for Hearing and Speech Action
10801 Rockville Pike
Rockville, MD 20852
(800) 638-8255

National Information Center on Deafness
Gallaudet University
800 Florida Ave. NE
Washington, DC 20002
(202) 651-5051

AT&T Special Needs Center
2001 Rte. 46, #310
Parsippany, NJ 07054
(800) 233-1222 (voice)
(800) 833-3232 (TDD)

Devices

American Communications Corp.
180 Roberts St.
East Hartford, CT 06108
(203) 289-3491 (voice/TDD)
>Baby criers, doorbell/phone signalers

AT&T National Speech Needs Center
2001 Rte. 46, #310
Parsippany, NJ 07054
(800) 233-1222 (voice)
(800) 833-3232 (TDD)
>Assistive listening devices, phone amplifiers, doorbell and phone signalers, answering machines, telecaption decoders, etc.

Audex
713 N. 4th St.
Longview, TX 75601
(800) 237-0716 (voice/TDD)
>Phone amplifiers

Audio Enhancement
8 Winfield Point Lane
St. Louis, MO 63141
(314) 367-6141
> Free information about wireless auditory assistance devices

Audiological Engineering Corp.
35 Medford St.
Somerville, MA 02143
(800) 238-4601
> Free information on infrared and loop-hearing systems and other assistive aids

G.N. Danavox, Inc.
6400 Flying Cloud Dr.
Eden Prairie, MN 55344
(612) 941-0690 (voice)
(800) 247-5343 (voice in Minnesota)
(800) 328-6297 (TDD)
> Phone amplifiers

Eye Festival, Inc.
1530 N. Gower St., Suite 201
Hollywood, CA 90028
(213) 873-3325 (voice)
(800) 873-3327 (TDD)
> Bed vibrators, wake-up alarms

General Technologies
7415 Windwing Way
Fair Oaks, CA 95628
(916) 962-9225 (voice/TDD)
> Free catalog, assistive listening devices

Hal-Hen Co.
35-53 24th St.
Long Island, NY 11106
(718) 392-6020
> Phone amplifiers, baby criers, doorbell/phone/fire/ smoke signalers, bed vibrators, wake-up alarms

Harris Communications
6541 City West Pkwy.
Eden Prairie, MN 55344
(800) 825-6758 (voice)
(800) 825-9187 (TDD)
> Free catalog, closed-caption and cable-ready decoder, TDDs, signalers, clocks, other devices

Hear You Are, Inc.
4 Musconetcong Ave.
Stanhope, NJ 07874
(201) 347-7662 (voice/TDD)
> Free catalog, doorbell signal, telephone aids, visual and smoke alarms, other assistive-listening devices

Independent Living Aids, Inc./Can-Do Products
27 East Mall
Plainview, NY 11803
(800) 537-2118
(516) 752-8080 (in New York)
> Free catalog, household items, communication aids

Julian McDermott Corp.
1639 Stephen St.
Ridgewood, NY 11385
(714) 456-3606 (voice)
> Burglar alarms, doorbell/fire/smoke signalers, wake-up alarms

National Captioning Institute, Inc.
5203 Leesburg Pike
Falls Church, VA 22041
(703) 845-1992
(703) 998-2400 (TDD)
    Free brochure, closed-captioned equipment

Nationwide Flashing Signal Systems
8120 Fenton St.
Silver Spring, MD 20910
(301) 589-6670 (TDD)
(301) 589-6671 (voice)
(301) 589-5153 (FAX)
    Free catalog, visual alerting devices including burglar
    alarms, baby criers, doorbell signalers, fire/smoke alarms,
    answering machines, pagers, phone signalers, telecaption
    decoders, bed vibrators, wake-up alarms, TDDs

One Video Place
405 Lowell St.
Wakefield, MA 01880
    Catalog $3.95, closed-captioned movies on videocassettes

Phone-TTY Inc.
202 Lexington Ave.
Hackensack, NJ 07601
(201) 489-7889
(201) 489-7890 (TDD)
    Free information, modems and software for using com-
    puters to talk with TDDS, baby criers, doorbell/fire/
    smoke signalers, wake-up alarms

Phonic Ear, Inc.
3880 Cypress Dr.
Petaluma, CA 94594
(800) 227-0735
(800) 772-3374 (in California)
    Free catalog, sound enhancers for group functions and
    personal FM systems

Potomac Technology
1 Church St., Suite 402
Rockville, MD 20850
(301) 762-4005
(301) 762-0851 (TDD)
    Free information, special-needs devices

Precision Controls, Inc.
14 Doty Rd.
Haskell, NJ 07420
(201) 835-5000 (voice/TDD)
    Baby criers, doorbell/fire/smoke/phone signalers, bed
    vibrators, wake-up alarms

Radio Shack
Division Tandy Corporation
One Tandy Center
Fort Worth, TX 76102
(817) 390-3011
    Free catalog, special-needs devices

Science Products
Box 888
Southeastern, PA 19399
(215) 296-2111
    Free catalog, voice sensory aids and electronics

Sennheiser
6 Vista Dr.
P.O. Box 987
Old Lyme, CT 06371
(203) 434-9190 (voice/TDD)
    Free information, easy-to-use transmitters and receivers
    with 16 selectable frequencies

Siemans Hearing Instruments, Inc.
10 Corporate Place South
Corporate Park 287
Piscataway, NJ 08854
(908) 562-6600
> Free information, easy-to-install infrared in-home TV listening system

Silent Call Corp.
P.O. Box 16348
Clarkson, MI 48016
(313) 391-1710
> Free information, electronically activated wireless personal alert system, baby criers, doorbell/fire/smoke/phone signalers

Sonic Alert, Inc.
1750 W. Hamlin
Rochester, MI 48309
(313) 656-3110 (voice/TDD)
> Baby criers, doorbell/fire/smoke/phone/signalers, bed vibrators, wake-up alarms

Sound Resources, Inc.
201 E. Ogden
Hinsdale, IL 60521
(708) 325-6133
> Assistive-listening devices

Tele-Consumer Hotline
1910 K. St. NW, Suite 610
Washington, DC 20006
(202) 223-4371 (voice/TDD)
(800) 332-1244
> Free information, assistive-listening devices

Temasek Telephone, Inc.
21 Airport Rd.
South San Francisco, CA 94080
(800) 647-8887
    Free information, voice-activated telephones

Ultratec
450 Science Dr.
Madison, WI 53711
(608) 238-5400
    Free catalog, all-in-one phone, baby criers, doorbell/fire/
    smoke/phone signalers, wake-up alarms

Weitbrecht Communications, Inc.
2656 29th St., Suite 205
Santa Monica, CA 90405
(800) 233-9130 (voice/TDD)
    Free catalog, assistive-listening devices and portable TDDs

Text Telephones (TT)/Telecommunications
Devices for the Deaf (TDD)

General Information
AT&T National Speech Needs Center
2001 Rte. 46, #310
Parsippany, NJ 07054
(800) 233-1222 (voice)
(800) 833-3232 (TDD)

National Center for Law and the Deaf
Gallaudet University
800 Florida Ave. NE
Washington, DC 20002
(202) 651-5373 (voice/TDD)
    Information on mandated state and federal relay systems

National Information Center on Deafness
Gallaudet University
800 Florida Ave. NE
Washington, DC 20002
(202) 651-5109 (voice)
(202) 651-5976 (TDD)

NTID
Dept. of Public Affairs
One Lomb Memorial Dr.
Rochester, NY 14623
    Brochure: "What You Should Know About TDDs"

Self-Help for Hard of Hearing People, Inc.
7800 Wisconsin Ave.
Bethesda, MD 20814
(301) 657-2248 (voice)
(301) 657-2249 (TDD)
    Brochure: "Beyond the Hearing Aid with Assistive Devices"

Telecommunications for the Deaf, Inc.
814 Thayer Ave.
Silver Spring, MD 20910
(301) 589-3786 (voice)
(301) 589-3006 (TDD)
    Directory: *International Telephone Directory of the Deaf*

Tele-Consumer Hotline
1910 K St. NW, Suite 610
Washington, DC 20006
(800) 332-1124 (voice/TDD)
(202) 223-4371 (voice/TDD)
    Chart: TDD relay center comparison chart

TT/TDD Devices
American Communications Corp.
180 Roberts St.
East Hartford, CT 06108
(203) 289-3491 (voice/TDD)

AT&T Information Products and Systems
60 Columbia Turnpike, Rm. A-A210
Morristown, NJ 07960
(800) 233-1222 (voice)
(800) 833-3232 (TDD)

Cascade Medical, Inc.
10180 Viking Dr.
Eden Prairie, MN 55344
(612) 941-7345

Deaf Communications of Cincinnati
550 Palmerston Dr.
Cincinnati, OH 45231
(513) 451-3722 (voice/TDD)

Guardian Communications Corp., Inc.
105 E. Annandale Rd., Suite 200
Falls Church, VA 22046
(703) 241-5805 (voice)

HARC Mercantile Ltd.
3130 Portage St.
P.O. Box 3055
Kalamazoo, MI 49003
    Voice synthesizers

Hearing Impaired Technology
Gallaudet University
P.O. Box 1742
800 Florida Ave. NE
Washington, DC 20002

IBM
National Support Center for Persons with Disabilities
P.O. Box 2150
Atlanta, GA 30055
(800) 426-2133 (voice)
(800) 284-9482 (TDD)

Integrated Microcomputer Systems, Inc.
2 Research Place
Rockville, MD 20850
(301) 948-4790 (voice)
(301) 869-6391 (TDD/ASCII 300)

International Technologies
Box 498
151 West Main St.
Duncan, SC 29334
    Echo 200, a TT-Touch-Tone phone system

Krown Research, Inc.
10371 W. Jefferson Blvd.
Culver City, CA 90232
(800) 883-4968 (outside CA only)
213-839-0181 (voice/TDD)

Nationwide Flashing Signal Systems
8120 Fenton St.
Silver Spring, MD 20910
(301) 589-6670 (TDD)
(301) 589-6671 (voice)
(301) 589-5153 (FAX)

Phone-TTY Inc.
202 Lexington Ave.
Hackensack, NJ 07601
(201) 489-7889
(201) 489-7890 (TDD)

Specialized Systems, Inc.
2525 Pioneer Ave., Suite 3
Vista, CA 92803
(800) 854-1559 (voice/TDD outside CA)
(619) 598-7337 (voice/TDD)

Ultratec
450 Science Dr.
Madison, WI 53711
(608) 238-5400

Zicom Technologies, Inc.
2485-A Coral St.
Vista, CA 92083
(800) 748-5633 (voice/TDD)
(619) 727-7110 (voice/TDD)

Hearing Ear Dog Programs

Hearing ear dogs can be any breed or size, and are usually obtained at humane shelters by a nonprofit training center. Many states have regional dog-training programs. For more information about hearing ear dogs, contact the following national programs:

American Humane Association
P.O. Box 1266
Denver, CO 80231
(303) 695-0811 (voice)
(303) 695-4531 (TDD)

Canine Companions for Independence
P.O. Box 446
Santa Rosa, CA 95402
(707) 528-0830

Canine Helpers for the Handicapped, Inc.
5705 Ridge Road
Lockport, NY 14904
(716) 433-4035 (voice/TDD)

Center for Hearing Ear Dogs
9725 E. Hampden Ave.
Denver, CO 80231
(303) 695-0811 (voice)
(303) 695-4531 (TDD)

Dogs for the Deaf, Inc.
110175 Wheeler Rd.
Central Point, OR 97502
(503) 899-7177 (voice)
(503) 846-6783 (TDD)

Hearing Ear Dog Program
P.O. Box 213
West Boylston, MA 01583
(508) 835-3304 (voice/TDD)

International Hearing Dogs, Inc.
5901 E. 89th Ave.
Henderson, CO 80640
(303) 287-3277 (voice/TDD)

National Hearing Dog Center
1116 S. Main
Athol, MA 01331
(508) 249-9264 (voice)

Red Acre Farm Hearing Dog Center
109 Red Acre Road
P.O. Box 278
Stow, MA 01775
(508) 897-5370 (voice)
(508) 897-8343 (TDD)

8

How to Adapt to a Hearing Loss

Learning how to adapt to a hearing loss can be a discouraging experience. Despite the growing number of hearing aids and assistive devices, the communication problems of those who are starting to have hearing problems can sometimes feel insurmountable. Still, there are ways you can improve communicating with others:

- Ask people to face you when they speak, and don't stand any farther away than three feet.
- If people continue to look away while they talk or place their hands over their faces, remind them politely to look at you directly.
- Don't assume friends will automatically remember what your communication needs are. If you can't hear well in certain situations, simply explain the problem briefly and suggest how they can help.
- At a meeting, sit where you can see the most people clearly.
- Sit at the head or foot of a table.

- Try to get an agenda or a copy of notes before a meeting if you anticipate problems in following along.
- Ask your friends to take notes for you.
- Ask in advance about the possibility of special listening devices, such as induction loops, radio-frequency hearing aids, or infrared systems.
- When attending the movies or a lecture, arrive early to get a good seat. Sit up front where you can best see and hear the speaker.
- At the movies, ask if there are devices available to amplify sound.

Adapting to a New Hearing Aid

One of the most difficult adaptations may well be handling your hearing aid. Research suggests that about 40 percent of consumers fitted with a hearing aid are dissatisfied with the result. Adjusting to a new hearing aid takes time and effort, just as a new pair of leather shoes must be broken in before they feel completely comfortable. One of the most common reasons that people end up with new hearing aids in their drawers is that they don't give themselves a chance to adapt to the devices before deciding they "don't work."

If you're getting ready to buy your first hearing aid, the first thing you need to realize is that your voice is going to sound quite different when you hear it the first time through a hearing aid. You have always heard your voice as it is filtered through the bones in your ear. When you hear your voice through a microphone in your hearing aid, it will sound to you the way your voice sounds on a tape recorder—like somebody else's voice entirely! When you first get your hearing aid, practice at home speaking out loud so you can get accustomed to your "new" voice.

Remember that not only will your own voice sound different—so will everyone else's. Your hearing aid is only a device to boost your ability to hear speech sounds; it can't hope to duplicate those sounds. Your hearing aid will change the quality of the tones you hear, making sounds clearer but also lending a mechanical, "tinny" sound. This can be annoying at first.

In many ways you'll have to learn how to hear all over again. You'll probably be surprised at all the new sounds you hear. Most likely you've been gradually losing your hearing for some time, and you have probably not realized the number of sounds you could no longer hear. With your new hearing aid you'll suddenly pick up your own breathing, a clock ticking, a bird singing. Although some of these sounds may be a pleasant surprise, others may become annoying or uncomfortable. Eventually you can learn to filter out unwanted sounds unconsciously using the same selective process that those with normal hearing perform thousands of times a day.

The key is not to become discouraged. No matter how annoying things get, try to avoid the temptation to remove your hearing aid when you get frustrated or annoyed. If you remove the aid every time things get rough, it will take longer to adapt.

However, you're just asking for trouble if you go out and get fitted with a new hearing aid and then wear it nonstop in all sorts of situations. Though it takes about an average of one to two weeks to adjust to a new aid, this period actually varies a great deal from one person to the next. Or, if you've been wearing aids for some time and you're now going in for a new set, don't expect the new aid to sound exactly like the old one—it won't.

Whether you're new to hearing aids or you've been wearing them for some time, when you get a new aid it's a good idea to set up a schedule for wearing the devices. Don't put them on immediately, but wait until you're relaxed at home where it's quiet and peaceful. Insert your aids and read out loud. Take them off and on, a little longer each time.

Start a conversation with one person. In a few days try conversations with several people. After a few more days you're ready to take a trip outside with the aids.

If Your Loved One Has a Hearing Problem . . .

If you have a relationship with someone who has experienced hearing loss—close friend, parent, spouse, child—you may think you understand their emotional responses. But odds are, you're both still struggling with the ways the person is responding to the loss. "So many of my friends don't understand why I need to sit in a corner of the restaurant away from the loudspeakers," complains Holly, 54. "They don't understand why I don't want to pay $7.50 to see a movie I can't hear. I don't want special treatment. I just wish people would understand what it's like."

Just as it may be hard for someone to accept encroaching hearing loss, it may also be hard for friends and family to accept that the person's hearing is getting worse. "I always knew that Betty was a little hard of hearing," recalls Karen, 43. "We were college roommates, and I'd have to repeat myself sometimes and speak louder on the phone. After we graduated and moved apart, she never discussed her hearing problem. I always assumed it was just a slight loss. But when we went out together to a restaurant and we had to change tables so that she could hear me, it finally hit me that she was more than just a little hard of hearing. That's when she told me she couldn't hear anything without her hearing aids. I guess my image of her had never changed from when we had been in college together."

Often family members accuse the hard-of-hearing person of manipulation: "You only hear what you want to hear," they say. Few things can make a person with a hearing loss angrier than this inaccurate statement.

Many people who have begun to lose their hearing report they often feel a range of emotions, including frustration, tension, fatigue, and fear of embarrassment. It's frustrating not to be able to understand normal conversation, to have to ask people to repeat themselves. Constantly feeling you must be alert to catch the drift of the conversation creates quite a bit of tension. You don't want to miss important points or lose the thread of the discussion altogether. All that alertness is enormously draining, requiring constant effort to fill in missed words and try to predict what's coming next. Finally, the fear of making an inappropriate comment fills some people with such anxiety that they stop interacting at all.

If you've ever been tempted to dismiss these feelings as overreactions, imagine how you would feel in similar circumstances. Anyone who has ever traveled to a foreign country and tried to communicate without being able to speak the language has encountered some of the same feelings.

"I remember being in France and trying to buy some fruit at a stand," recalls Tim, whose friend Peter has a serious hearing problem. "I didn't speak any French, and I was trying to find out how much everything cost. There was a big line behind me, and I had to keep asking the grocer to repeat himself. He was getting more arrogant by the second. He kept rolling his eyes and making remarks to the others behind me in French. Everybody else was laughing, and I knew they were laughing at me. That's the way I think it must be for Peter sometimes when he tries to communicate with people who hear more than he does."

Sometimes people with a hearing problem report being treated as if they were mentally inferior. "People treat [my husband] as if he was the village idiot because he can't hear," complains Jean, 45. Her husband, a brilliant astrophysicist, has problems with his self-confidence in the face of others' rejection.

The tension that's generated by struggling to follow the

thread of a conversation when only half of the words make any sense can be profoundly exhausting. If you've ever been 10 minutes late for an extremely important meeting, you'll know how draining tension can be. Imagine you're on your way to an important business presentation and you're backed up in traffic that isn't moving. Every second that ticks by seems like an eternity. You can actually feel the pressure build, pounding in your temples. By the time you arrive at your meeting, you probably feel like collapsing, totally exhausted. You haven't *physically* been doing anything more strenuous than sitting behind the wheel of a car—but the *emotional* strain can leave you exhausted.

Then there is the fear of embarrassment at making an inappropriate comment. Think how it would feel to walk into a party filled with royalty or heads of state. Everyone is chatting knowledgeably, and you're filled with nervousness at the thought of making an inappropriate comment.

This is why communication with hearing friends or family members can be seen as simply too much effort by someone with a hearing loss, and why sometimes he withdraws from social situations completely. Of course, it can also be frustrating for friends and family members to try to communicate.

"It's awful," sighed Tanya, 46, whose husband has a hearing problem. "He can't hear what you say, and he keeps saying, 'What?' We had a big argument about the TV the other day, because he kept asking me what was going on."

Tips on Communication

There are several things to keep in mind when communicating with someone who is hard of hearing.

Get the person's attention. Before you start speaking, make sure the person who is hard of hearing is paying attention; call her name or touch her. By watching your face, she can deduce valuable cues to help in understanding your words.

Decrease background noise. It's very difficult for a person with a hearing problem to understand conversation if there is lots of other competing noises in the background—other people talking, dogs barking, stereos playing. Turn off the TV set or radio and close the windows if there is outside traffic noise. If you can't avoid background noise, try moving to a quieter area.

Move in closer. Especially in the presence of background noise, move within two to three feet of the person with whom you are talking so that your speech will be louder than other distracting noises. Don't talk from another room.

Don't shout. Remember to keep your speech at a normal level if the person is wearing a hearing aid. If the person isn't and you know he has a hearing problem, you can speak a little louder than normal, but don't shout.

Speak normally. Try to speak naturally; don't slow your speech to the point that it seems insulting. Pause more often. If you're a naturally fast speaker, try to slow down, since rapid speech is more difficult to follow.

Articulate. Speak clearly and articulate well, but don't exaggerate your mouth movements.

Hold still. Don't make lots of gestures or move your head around, which can be distracting.

Be alert. While communicating, be aware of slight facial nuances that might mean the person is not understanding what you are saying. Many people who are hard of hearing will sometimes nod as if they understand you to avoid having to keep asking you to repeat yourself.

Watch pitch. Keep the pitch of your conversation fairly low, since a lower-pitched voice is easier to understand. Don't mumble.

Concentrate. Don't do other things at the same time you're talking, and don't talk when you're distracted.

Gestures. Use appropriate body language and facial expressions.

If the person to whom you're speaking doesn't understand you, don't say, "Turn up your hearing aid!" or accuse the person of paying attention only when it pleases her. In the first place, many people with hearing loss (especially age-related) often hear speech as distorted. Turning up the volume on a hearing aid can't make distorted sound any clearer; it can actually make it worse. It can also be painful. If you haven't been understood, try these suggestions:

- Repeat the sentence using the same words ("Where's my purse?").
- Try to rephrase the sentence with different words ("Have you seen my handbag?").
- Break up your sentence into two phrases ("I need my pocketbook. Do you know where it is?").
- Write down the key words.
- Make sure you're looking at the person and speaking clearly.

Remember that even if your loved one is fairly good at speechreading (reading lips), almost no one can follow a complete conversation just by using this method. At best, speechreading can give a person *clues* about what is being said. Too many speech sounds can't be detected by reading the lip movements, and too many words look identical when spoken.

Modern technology has made great strides in the

development of powerful hearing aids that are almost invisible. In addition, a wide range of assistive systems and alerting devices may also help your loved one's communication problems.

Appendix

Organizations and Resources

Alexander Graham Bell Association for the Deaf
3417 Volta Place NW
Washington, DC 20007
(202) 337-5220 (voice/TDD)

American Association of the Deaf-Blind
814 Thayer Ave., 3rd Fl.
Silver Spring, MD 20910
(301) 588-6545

American Academy of Otolaryngology—Head and Neck
  Surgery
One Prince St.
Alexandria, VA 22316
(703) 836-4444 (voice)

American Athletic Association of the Deaf, Inc.
1052 Darling St.
Ogden, UT 84403
(801) 393-8710

American Deafness and Rehabilitation Association
P.O. Box 55369
Little Rock, AR 72225
(501) 663-7074 (voice/TDD)

American Hearing Research Foundation
55 E. Washington St., Suite 2022
Chicago, IL 60602
(312) 726-9670 (voice)

American Society for Deaf Children
814 Thayer Ave., 3rd Fl.
Silver Spring, MD 20910
(301) 585-5400 (voice/TDD)

American Society of Deaf Social Workers
c/o Mental Health Services for Hearing Impaired Persons
Horizon Hospital
11200 U.S. 19th S
Clearwater, FL 33546
(813) 541-2646 (voice/TDD)

American Speech-Language-Hearing Association
10801 Rockville Pike
Rockville, MD 20852
(301) 897-5700 (voice/TDD)
(800) 897-8682 (helpline)

American Tinnitus Association
P.O. Box 5
Portland, OR 97207
(503) 248-9985 (voice)

Association of Late-Deafened Adults
1027 Oakton
Evanston, IL 60202

Better Hearing Institute
P.O. Box 1840
Washington, DC 20013
(800) EAR-WELL (voice)
(703) 642-0580 (voice)

The Caption Center
125 Western Ave.
Boston, MA 02134
(617) 492-9225 (voice/TDD)

Captioned Films for the Deaf
5000 Park St. N
St. Petersburg, FL 33709
(800) 237-6213 (voice/TDD)

Center for Bicultural Studies, Inc.
5506 Kenilworth Ave., Suite 105
Riverdale, MD 20737
(301) 277-3945

Center on Deafness
10100 Dee Rd.
Des Plaines, IL 60016
(708) 297-1022

Children of Deaf Adults
c/o Texas School for the Deaf
P.O. Box 3538
Austin, TX 78764
(512) 440-5300

Cochlear Implant Club International
P.O. Box 464
Buffalo, NY 14223
(716) 838-4662 (voice/TDD)

Cochlear Implant Information Center
61 Inverness Dr. East, Suite 200
Englewood, CO 80112
(800) 458-4999 (voice/TDD except Colorado)
(301) 790-9010 (voice/TDD in Colorado)

Conference of Educational Administrators Serving the Deaf
    American School for the Deaf
139 N. Main St.
West Hartford, CT 06107
(203) 727-1304 (voice/TDD)

Convention of American Instructors of the Deaf
P.O. Box 2025
Austin, TX 78768
(512) 441-2225 (voice/TDD)

D.E.A.F., Inc.
215 Brighton Ave.
Allston, MA 02134
(617) 254-4041 (voice/TDD)

Deaf Artists of America
87 N. Clinton Ave., Suite 408
Rochester, NY 14604
(716) 325-2400 (voice/TDD)

Deafness Research Foundation
9 E. 38th St.
New York, NY 10016
(212) 684-6556 (voice)
(212) 684-6559 (TDD)
(800) 535-DEAF

DEAFPRIDE, Inc.
1350 Potomac Ave. SE
Washington, DC 20003
(202) 675-6700 (voice/TDD)

Deaf Women United
215 Brighton Ave.
Allston, MA 02134
(617) 254-4041 (voice/TDD)

The Ear Foundation
(The Menière's Network)
2000 Church St.
Box 111
Nashville, TN 37326
(800) 545-HEAR (voice/TDD)

Gallaudet Research Institute
800 Florida Ave. NE
Washington, DC 20002
(202) 651-5400
(800) 451-8834

Genetic Service Center
Gallaudet Research Institute
Gallaudet University
800 Florida Ave. NE
Washington, DC 20002
(202) 651-5258 (voice/TDD)
(800) 672-6720, x 5258 (voice/TDD)

Hearing Industries Association
1800 M St. NW
Washington, DC 20036
(202) 833-1411

Hear Now
4001 S. Magnolia Way, Suite 100
Denver, CO 80237
(800) 648-HEAR (voice/TDD)

Helen Keller National Center for Deaf-Blind Youths and
Adults
111 Middle Neck Rd.
Sands Point, NY 11050
(516) 944-8900 (voice/TDD)

House Ear Institute
256 S. Lake
Los Angeles, CA 90057
(213) 483-4431 (voice)
(213) 484-2642 (TDD)

International Association of Parents of the Deaf
814 Thayer Ave., 3rd Fl.
Silver Spring, MD 20910
(301) 588-6545

International Foundation for Children's Hearing, Education,
and Research
871 McLean Ave.
Yonkers, NY 10704

Junior National Association of the Deaf Youth Programs
445 N. Pennsylvania St., Suite 804
Indianapolis, IN 46204
(301) 587-1788 (voice/TDD)

National Association for Hearing and Speech Action
10801 Rockville Pike
Rockville, MD
(800) 638-TALK (voice/TDD)

National Association of the Deaf
814 Thayer Ave., 3rd Fl.
Silver Spring, MD 20910
(301) 587-1788 (voice/TDD)

National Black Deaf Advocates, Inc.
P.O. Box 91166
Washington, DC 20066
(301) 559-5398 (TDD)

National Captioning Institute, Inc.
5203 Leesburg Pike
Falls Church, VA 22041
(703) 998-2400 (voice/TDD)

National Center for Law and the Deaf
Gallaudet University
800 Florida Ave. NE
Washington, DC 20002
(202) 651-5373 (voice/TDD)

National Crisis Center for the Deaf
University of Virginia Medical Center
P.O. Box 484
Charlottesville, VA 29087
(800) 552-7917 (inside Virginia, voice/TDD)

National Cued Speech Association
P.O. Box 31345
Raleigh, NC 27622
(919) 828-1218 (voice/TDD)

National Foundation for Children's Hearing Education and
    Research
928 McLean Ave.
Yonkers, NY 10704
(914) 237-2676

National Fraternal Society of the Deaf
1300 W. Northwest Hwy.
Mt. Prospect, IL 60056
(312) 392-9282 (voice)
(312) 392-1409 (TDD)
(800) 876-NFSD (voice/TDD)

National Hearing Aid Society
20361 Middlebelt
Livonia, MI 48152
(313) 478-2610 (voice)
(800) 521-5247 (helpline)

National Hearing Association
1010 Jorie Blvd., Suite 308
Oak Brook, IL 60521
(312) 323-7200

National Information Center for Children and Youth with
  Handicaps
P.O. Box 1492
Washington, DC 20013
(703) 893-6061 (voice/TDD)
(800) 999-5599

National Information Center on Deafness
Gallaudet College
800 Florida Ave. NE
Washington, DC 20002
(202) 651-5051 (voice)
(202) 651-5052 (TDD)

National Rehabilitation Information Center
8455 Colesville Rd., Suite 935
Silver Spring, MD 20910
(301) 588-9284 (voice/TDD)
(800) 34-NARIC

National Research Register for Hereditary Hearing Loss
Boys Town National Research Hospital
555 30th St.
Omaha, NE 68154
(402) 498-6631 (voice/TDD)

The National Theatre of the Deaf
P.O. Box 659
Chester, CT 06412
(203) 526-4971 (voice)
(203) 526-4974 (TDD)

Parmly Hearing Institute
Loyola University of Chicago
6525 N. Sheridan Rd.
Chicago, IL 60626
(312) 508-2710

Project ALAS
c/o D.E.A.F., Inc.
215 Brighton Ave.
Allston, MA 02134
(617) 254-4041 (voice/TDD)

Quota International, Inc.
1420 21st St. NW
Washington, DC 20036
(202) 331-9694 (voice/TDD)

Rainbow Alliance of the Deaf
P.O. Box 14182
Washington, DC 20044
(202) 779-6459 (TDD)

Registry of Interpreters for the Deaf, Inc.
511 Monroe St., Suite 1107
Rockville, MD 20850
(301) 779-0555 (voice/TDD)

The See Center for the Advancement of Deaf Children
P.O. Box 1181
Los Alamitos, CA 90720
(310) 430-1467

Self-Help for Hard of Hearing People, Inc. (SHHH)
7800 Wisconsin Ave.
Bethesda, MD 20814
(301) 657-2248 (voice)
(301) 657-2249 (TDD)

Sign Instructors Guidance Network (SIGN)
814 Thayer Ave.
Silver Spring, MD 20910
(301) 587-1788

Telecommunications for the Deaf, Inc.
814 Thayer Ave.
Silver Spring, MD 20910
(301) 589-3786 (voice)
(301) 589-3006 (TDD)

Tele-Consumer Hotline
1910 K St. NW, Ste. 610
Washington, DC 20006
(202) 223-4371 (voice/TDD)
(800) 332-1124 (voice/TDD outside D.C.)

TRIPOD
2901 N. Keystone St.
Burbank, CA 91504
(800) 352-8888
(800) 346-8888 (California only)
(818) 972-2080 (voice/TDD)

U.S. Deaf Skiers Association
Box USA
Gallaudet University
800 Florida Ave. NE
Washington, DC 20002
(202) 651-5255 (TDD)

Vestibular Disorders Association of America
1015 NW 22nd Ave., D230
Portland, OR 97120
(503) 229-7705 (voice)

World Recreation Association of the Deaf, Inc./USA
P.O. Box 321
Quartz Hill, CA 93586
(800) 342-5833 (voice relay; California only)
(805) 943-8879 (TDD)

Glossary

acoustic Pertaining to sound or the sense of hearing.

acoustic nerve See *auditory nerve.*

adenoids The two lymph nodes above the tonsils at the back of the nose that are partly responsible for protecting the body's upper respiratory tract against infection.

air conduction Transmission of sound to the inner ear by way of the ear canal and the middle ear.

air-bone gap The difference in decibels between the hearing threshold levels for a particular frequency as determined by air conduction and bone conduction. This difference is used to help determine the type of treatment a person needs.

anvil The middle of the three bones (ossicles) in the middle ear that transmits sound vibrations.

audiologist A person with a degree and/or certification in the areas of identification and measurement of hearing impairments and rehabilitation of those with hearing problems.

audiology The study of the entire field of hearing, including the nature and conservation of hearing, identification and assessment of hearing loss, and the rehabilitation of all those with hearing impairments.

auditory nerve The part of the eighth cranial nerve that carries information from the inner ear to the brain. It consists of two separate divisions, the vestibular nerve and the cochlear nerve. The auditory nerve is also called the acoustic nerve or the hearing nerve.

auditory perception The mental awareness of sound.

auditory training The process of teaching a person with hearing loss to take full advantage of any sound cues that can still be heard. Like speechreading, auditory training can help those with hearing loss become aware of cues they might not otherwise notice. The type of auditory training depends on when the person lost hearing and the type of hearing loss.

auricle The outer part of the external ear, also called the pinna.

basilar membrane A flexible membrane that is attached to the bony shelf and divides the coil of the cochlea lengthwise into two compartments; as sounds disturb the perilymph fluid on one side of the membrane, they are transferred through the basilar membrane to the organ of Corti on the other side, and on to the hair cells.

bone conduction The process by which sound is transmitted to the inner ear through the bones of the skull.

central hearing loss A type of hearing loss caused by damage or impairment in the nerves or nuclei of the central nervous system, either in the pathways to the brain or in the brain itself.

cerumen Brown ear wax secreted into the external ear canal.

closed-captioned TV A line of printed text of the conversations that appears on a TV screen during certain programs when an adaptor is attached to the TV.

cochlea The hearing part of the inner ear. This snail-shaped structure contains fluid and thousands of microscopic hair cells tuned to various frequencies, in addition to the organ of Corti (the receptor for hearing).

conductive hearing loss A hearing deficit caused by a problem in the middle or outer ear.

decibel Measure of the intensity (loudness) of sound.

digitally programmable hearing aid A hearing aid for which the characteristics are set and adjusted via microcomputer, allowing more specific fitting and flexibility.

discrimination This refers to the ability to understand speech once it is loud enough to hear.

eardrum A paper-thin covering stretching across the ear canal that separates the middle and the outer ears.

ENT specialist A physician who specializes in the treatment of problems associated with the ear, nose, and throat. This is another name for otolaryngologist or head and neck surgeon.

eustachian tube The air duct that connects the area behind the nose to the middle ear.

frequency A measure of the pitch of a sound.

hair cells Sensory receptors in the inner ear that transform sound vibrations into the messages traveling to the brain.

inner ear The interior section of the ear, where sound vibrations and information about balance are translated into nerve impulses.

middle ear The small cavity between the eardrum and the oval window that houses the three tiny bones of hearing (the ossicles).

nerve deafness The former term for sensorineural hearing loss.

ossicles The three small bones of the middle ear (the malleus or hammer, the incus or anvil, and the stapes or stirrup). These bones help carry sound and speech from the eardrum to the inner ear.

otologist A physician specialist primarily interested in diagnosing ear diseases, specifying causes of hearing loss, and treating physical defects of the auditory mechanism. Otology is a division of the ear, nose, and throat field (otolaryngology).

otoscope An instrument used for examining the ear, to inspect the outer ear canal and the eardrum, and to detect certain diseases of the middle ear.

outer ear The portion of the ear that contains the external ear (or pinna).

oval window A tiny opening in the body wall of the cochlea that is an entrance to the inner ear.

pinna The part of the outer ear that we can see, also called the auricle.

presbycusis A type of progressive sensorineural hearing loss associated with aging; it is one of the most common chronic problems among older people.

pure tone A sound at only one frequency (pitch) with no harmonics.

recruitment An abnormal, rapid increase in loudness as the strength of the acoustic signal is increased.

resonance The vibration of an object or air when certain pitches are made louder (such as when a person blows over the top of a bottle).

semicircular canals Another name for the labyrinth, the organ inside the inner ear that is connected to the cochlea but does not contribute to the sense of hearing. Instead these three fluid-filled loops help maintain balance by sending information about the position of the head along the auditory nerve to the brain.

sensorineural hearing loss A type of hearing loss that is caused by damage to the hair cells of the inner ear or the nerves that supply it. It is unlike conductive hearing loss, which is caused by diseases or obstructions in the outer or middle ear.

speech-language pathologist (speech therapist) A specialist in human communication, its development, and its disorders. This expert evaluates and treats those with communication problems resulting from total or partial hearing loss, brain injury, cleft palate, voice pathology, emotional problems, foreign dialect, development delays, stroke, learning disabilities, and so forth. They also provide clinical therapy to help those with speech and language disorders, and help them and their families understand the disorder and develop better communication skills.

stapedectomy An operation to treat hearing loss caused by otosclerosis in which all or most of the stapes are replaced by a plastic prosthesis.

stirrup The common term for the stapes, one of the three ossicles in the middle ear.

telecommunication device for the deaf (TDD) This visual typewriter device allows people to send typed phone messages over the telephone network. This generic term replaces the earlier term TTY, which refers specifically to teletypewriter machines.

tinnitus Often called ringing in the ears, this term refers to a ringing, buzzing, hissing, or whistling noise heard inside the ear when the acoustic nerve transmits impulses to the brain—

impulses produced not from outside vibrations, but as the result of stimuli produced inside the head.

tympanum The main part of the middle ear cavity that lies between the tympanic membrane and the lateral bony wall of the internal ear.

vestibule A portion of the labyrinth of the inner ear located between the cochlea and the semicircular canals.

INDEX

Acoustic, 156
Acoustic-immitance test, 19–20
Acoustic neuroma, 10
Acoustic-reflex test, 20
Adenoids, 31, 32, 156
Adults
  causes of hearing loss in,
    45–60
  and conductive hearing loss,
    9
  symptoms of hearing loss in,
    2
Age-related hearing loss, 1,
    45–48
  and sensorineural hearing
    loss, 10–11
  warning signs of, 47
  See also Presbycusis
AIDS, 54–55
Air-bone gap, 18, 156

Air conduction, 156
Air-pressure change test, 20
Alarm clocks, 107
Alcohol, 28, 60
Alerting devices, 107–10
  doorbell ringers, 108
  telephone ring alternatives,
    110
  visual alarms, 108–09
  vibrator alarms, 109–10
  where to get, 123, 125–30
Alexander Graham Bell
    Association for the
    Deaf, 47, 48
Allergies, 52
Alport's disease, 40
American Academy of
    Pediatrics, 34
American Society of Human
    Genetics, 43

American Speech Language
   Hearing Association, 15
Amikacin, 28, 58
Aminoglycosides, 28, 58, 59
Amoxicillin, 32
Amplified microphone,
   111–13
Amplifier
   hearing aid, 74–75
      K-amp type, 88
      programmable, 85, 88
   TV, 117
   telephone handset, 116–17
AM receiver headset, 113
Anemia, 48
Anoxia, 27
Answering machines, 122–23,
   127
Antibiotics
   as cause of hearing loss,
      58–59
   for ear problems, 31–32,
      51
Anti-cancer drugs, 60
Antihistamines, 32, 52
Antrum, 50
Anvil, 5–6, 62, 156
APGAR rating, 41
ARC patients, 54
ASCII code, 122
Aspirin, 59
Assistive listening systems,
   98–99, 107, 110–14
   DAI, 111
   extension microphones,
      111–13
   how to get information on,
      123–35

induction, 110–11
infrared systems, 114
where to get, 124–30
See also Telecommunications
   devices for the deaf
   (TDD); Telephone
   aids; Television aids;
   Text-telephones (TT)
Atherosclerosis, 10
Atropine, 52
Attachable portable amplifier,
   116
AT&T Special Needs Center,
   124, 130
Audio induction loop, 118
Audiologist, 15–16, 47, 77–78,
   156
   and hearing aid selection,
      75–76
   testing and evaluation by,
      15–20
   where to find, 16
Audiology, 157
Auditory brainstem response
   test (ABR), 41–42
Auditory "hearing" nerve
   defined, 5, 6, 157
   problems, 10, 30
Auditory neuritis, 48
Auditory perception, 157
Auditory training, 15, 157
Auricle. See Pinna
Automatic gain, 89
Automatic signal processing, 89
Autosomal dominant
   inheritance, 39
Autosomal recessive
   inheritance, 38–39

Baby criers, 124–30
Background noise
    and communication, 142
    and hearing aids, 83–85, 87,
        88
Bacterial infections
    and childhood deafness,
        30–33
    and prenatal hearing loss,
        25
Bacterial labyrinthitis, 50
Balance, 6–7
    tests, 15
Barbiturates, 52
Barotrauma, 9
Basilar membrane, 157
Battery, 97, 98
Baudot code, 122
Behind-the-ear hearing aid,
        76, **93**
    caring for, 97
    cost of, 81
    defined, 92–93
Better Hearing Institute, 123
Bi-CROS system aid, 94
Bilirubin, 26–27
Binaural hearing aids, 95
Birth injury, 41
Blockage, 9
Blood pooling, 57
Blood transfusions, 24, 27
Blood vessels, 5
Bone conduction, 18, 157
Bone-conduction hearing aids,
        92
Brain
    abscess, 49, 50
    hearing center, 10

Bumetanide, 59
Burglar alarms, 126

Cable TV, 118, 119–20
Caesar, Julius, 66
Caffeine, 60
Canal aid, **90**, 90–91
Carbon monoxide, 60
Cartilage, **5**
Cats, 23
CCC-A (Clinical Certificate of
        Competence—
        Audiology), 15
Cefixime, 32
Central hearing loss, 11, 157
Cerebral palsy (CP), 27
Cerumen, 157
Chemotherapy, 60
Chickenpox, 34
Children, 21–44
    acquired deafness in, 30–37,
        50
    and cochlear implants,
        101–03, 104–06
    and conductive hearing loss,
        9
    detecting hearing loss in,
        29, 36–37
    and hearing aids, 74, 95
    hereditary deafness, 38–40
    prenatal hearing loss in,
        21–29
    and sensorineural hearing
        loss, 10
    symptoms in, 2
    testing, 19–20
Chloroquine, 60
Cholesteatoma, 49, 50

Chromosomes, 38
Circulation problems, 11
Closed-caption TV, 118,
        119–20
    decoders, 126, 127
    movies on videocassette, 127
Cochlea, 56
    and age, 46
    and bone conduction, 18
    defined, 5, 6, 158
    drugs toxic to, 58
    meningeal labyrinthitis, 50
    and noise, 63
    and otosclerosis, 53
    testing, 58
Cochlear implants, 11, 99,
        101–05
    FDA regulations on, 104
Cochlear Menière's disease, 51
Cogan's syndrome, 40
Cohen, Dr. Noel, 105
Communication
    improving with normal
        hearing friends, 136–37
    with someone who's hard of
        hearing, 141–44
Communication aids, 107
Compression, 89
Compression circuits, 99
Computers, 122–23, 127
Conductive hearing loss, 9,
        158
    and injury, 57
    and otosclerosis, 53, 54
    test for, 18
Configuration of hearing loss,
        7, 8

Congenital hearing loss,
        20–29, 38
Congenital syphilis, 26
Conjunctivitis, 32
Consonants, 8, 10
Conversations, 46. *See also*
        Communication
Counseling, 17
CROS (crossover system) aid,
        94
CT scan, 103
Cysplatin, 60
Cytomegalovirus (CMV), 22,
        23–25, 41, 55

Day care, 24, 25
Deaf community, and cochlear
        implant controversy,
        102
Deaf parents, 39
Decibels (dB)
    danger zone, 63–64, 65
    defined, 6, 158
    and degree of hearing loss,
        7–8
Decongestants, 32
Deformity, 4
Degree of hearing ability, 7–8,
        17
Diabetes, 10, 55
Diagnosis, 13, 17
    of children, 29
    guidelines for, 13–14
    of infants, 41–42
Diet, 52
Digital hearing aid, 76
    add-ons, 89
    cost of, 81, 89

defined, 84–88, 158
manufacturers, 86–87
Direct audio input (DAI), 111
    and personal FM system, 112
    and TV, 118
Discrimination score, 19, 158
Distortion, 83
Diuretics, 28, 59
Dizziness, 4, 14
    and balance, 6
    and head injury, 56
    and Menière's disease, 51
DNA, 38
Doctor, 14–15, 74. *See also*
    ENT physician
Dominant genes, 39
Doorbell ringers, **108**, 124–30
Drainage, 4, 14
Drugs, 10, 11, 38
    deafness caused by, 22, 28,
        41, 57–60

Ear abscesses, 33
Earache, 31
Ear canal, 4–5
Ear diseases and infections, 9
    and adult hearing loss,
        48–54
    and bacterial labyrinthitis,
        50
    and childhood hearing loss,
        30–32
    and prenatal hearing loss,
        25–26
Eardrum (tympanum)
    and cholesteatoma, 49
    and conductive hearing loss,
        9

defined, 4–5, 158, 161
relieving pressure, 32
ruptured, 9, 57, 62
testing, 20
Earlens, 96
Earmold
    and behind-the-ear aids, 92
    custom-fitted vs. ready-
        made, 75
    discomfort, 100–01
    sensitivity to, 80
Earmuffs, 67, 69
Earplugs, 67, 68–69
Ear protectors, 65, 67–68
Ears
    balance mechanism, 6–7
    hearing mechanism, 4–6
Ear wax
    build-up, 4, 46
    guard, 97
    and hearing aid, 100–01
Easter Seals Society, 82
Emphysema, 10
Encephalitis, 27, 34, 35
Endocrine problems, 52
ENT (ear, nose, and throat)
    physician, 14, 20, 158
Environmental Protection
    Agency, 67
Ephedrine nose drops, 32
Ethacrynic acid, 28
Eustachian tube
    and air pressure
        equalization, 7
    defined, **5**, 158
    and balance mechanism, 7
    and childhood hearing loss,
        30, 31

Eustachian tube (*cont.*)
  and cholesteatoma, 49
  and conductive hearing loss,
    9
Extension microphones,
  111–13
External blockage, 36
Eyeglass hearing aid models,
  94
Eythacrynic acidrythromycin,
  58–59

Fatigue, 3
Federal Aviation Act (1968),
  66
Federal Aviation Agency, 67
Feedback, 99
  and telephone, 116
Fetal alcohol syndrome, 28
Fetal distress, 41
Fever, 11, 31
FM system, 113
Food and Drug
    Administration, 14
  cochlear implant
    regulations, 104
  hearing aid regulations, 74
Frequency
  defined, 158
  and degree of hearing loss,
    8, 10, 45–46
  and digital hearing aids, 85,
    88
  and pure-tone air-
    conduction test, 17
  and range of hearing aid, 84
Friends and family members
  with hearing problems

communicating with,
    141–44
  emotions of, 139–41
Full concha, 88
Fullness, 51, 62
Functional hearing loss, 11–12
Functional overlay, 12
Furosemide, 28, 59

Gain, 84, 89
Gallaudet Research Institute,
    Genetic Services
    Center, 42, 43
Genetic (hereditary) hearing
    problems, 10, 28
  causes of, 38–40
  diagnosing, 41–42
  resources, 42, 43–44
Gentamicin, 28, 58
German measles. *See* Rubella
Glucose tolerance problems,
  52
Group B Streptococcus, 25–26

Hair cells, 6, 158
  and age, 45–46
  and noise, 62, 63, 64
Half-concha, 88
Hammer, 5–6, 62
Hard-wired microphones, 112
Hard-wired TV devices, 117
Head injury, 10, 11, 27, 56–57
"Head shadow," 94
Hearing-aid compatible
    (HAC) telephone, 115
Hearing aid dealer or
    specialist
  vs. audiologist, 16

job of, 79–80
legal obligations of, 14
licensing, 77
Hearing aid evaluation, 15,
    71–72, 75–76
  test, 17
Hearing aid(s), 47, 71–106
  adapting to new, 137–39
  add-ons, 89
  adjusting, 80
  and assistive listening
      systems, 110–14
  basic service package, 80–81
  batteries, 91, 92, 97, 98
  breakdown of, 100–01
  caring for, 96–97
  cost of, 77, 78, 79, 81, 89
  FDA regulations, 74
  features, 98–100
    compression circuits, 99
    high-frequency aids, 99
    implantable aids, 99–100
    noise-reduction circuits,
        99
    T-coil and switch, 98
  finding dealer, 77–79
  fitting, 79–80
  help in paying for, 82
  how to buy, 14, 79–81
  how to get information on,
      106
  mail order, 77
  main characteristics, 84
  modern, 74–75
  problems with, 101
  pros and cons of, 72–73
  and sensorineural hearing
      loss, 10

and social stigma, 2
and telephone, 114–17
trial period and warranty,
    79, 81
types of, 83–96
  behind-the-ear, 76, 81, **93**,
      92–93, 97
  CROS, 94
  digital, 76, 81, 83–89, 158
  eyeglass, 94
  in-the-canal, **90**, 90–91, 99
  in-the-ear, 81, 88, **91**, 99
  K-amp, 88, 89
  magnetic, 96
  minaural/binaural, 95
  on-the-body, 76, 95
"Hearing ear" dog, 107,
    134–35
Hearing evaluation, 17, 20
Hearing loss
  adapting to, 136–44
  age-related, 1, 10–11, 45–48
  causes of
    acquired in childhood,
        30–38
    and drugs, 57–60
    hereditary, 38–44
    and infectious diseases, in
        adults, 45–56
    and injuries, 56–57
    and noise, 61–70
    prenatal, 21–29
    work-related, 64–65
  communication tips for,
      136–37, 141–44
  configuration of, 7
  defined, 1–2
  degree of, 7–8

Hearing loss (*cont.*)
  diagnosis of, 17
    in adults, 13–20
    in children, 29
    in infants, 41–42
    in friends and family
      members, 139–44
  organizations and resources
    for, 145–55
  medical correction of, 20
  symptoms of, 2–4
    in children, 36–37
  types of, 7, 9–12
    central, 11, 157
    conductive, 9, 18, 53, 54,
      57, 158
    functional or
      psychogenic, 11–12, 42
    mild, 7
    mixed, 11
    moderate, 7
    profound, 8
    sensorineural, 9–11,
      23–24, 26, 28, 33, 50,
      54, 160
    severe, 7–8
  tests for, 15–20
Hearing mechanism, 4–6
Hearing tests, 15, 16–20
  auditory brainstem response
    (ABR), 41–42
  getting results, 78
  pure bone conduction, 18
  pure-tone air-conduction,
    17–18
  speech-reception, 17, 18–19
Hear Now, 82
Heart problems, 10

Herpes simplex, 22, 23, 35, 41
Herpes zoster, 34, 35
H. flu, 32
Hib vaccine, 33
High-frequency aids, 99
High-pitched sounds, 10
HIV infection, 54
House Ear Institute, 52
Hydroxychloroquine, 60
Hypoxia, 27

IBM Phone Communicator,
  122
Implantable aids, 99–100. *See
  also* Cochlear implants
Incus. *See* Anvil
Indapamide, 59
Indifference, 3
Induction systems, 110–11,
  137
Infant apnea, 41
Infections, and prenatal
  hearing loss, 25–26
Influenza, 22, 25
Infrared listening system, **113**,
  137
  defined, 114
  for TV, 118
  where to get, 125
Injury, 56–57
Inner ear, 4, 56
  defined, **5**, 6, 158
  infections, 30, 33
  and sensorineural hearing
    loss, 9–11
  testing sensitivity of, 18
Insecurity, 3
Insulin, 52

Intermittent hearing loss, 36
In-the-canal (CIC) aid, **90**,
        90–91
    and telecoil, 99
In-the-ear aid
    cost of, 81
    defined, 88, **91**
    and telecoil, 99
Isolation, 1

Jaundice, 27, 41
Jet engine mechanics, 63–64
Job
    ear protectors for, 67–69
    reducing noise on, 69–70
    risky environments, 64–67

K-amp hearing aid, 88, 89
Kanamycin, 28, 41, 58
Kidney problems, 10, 28,
        55–56

Labor Department, 67
Labyrinthitis, 48, 49–50
Light timer, 107
Loop diuretics, 59
Loop-hearing systems, 125. *See
        also* Induction systems
Lyme disease, 55

Magnetic aids, 96
Malleus. *See* Hammer
March of Dimes Birth Defects
        Foundation, 43
Marsters, James, 121
Mastoid bone, 50
Mastoidectomy, 49, 51
Mastoiditis, 33, 50–51

Maximum power output, 83
Measles, 34–35
Medicaid, 82
Menière's disease, 10, 51–53
Meningeal labyrinthitis, 50
Meninges, 49
Meningitis, 25, 27, 33, 49, 50
Microphone, hearing aid, 74
Microsurgery, 57
Middle ear, 4, **5**, 158
    and childhood hearing loss,
        30–31
    and conductive hearing loss,
        9
    and infections, 49
    and injury, 57
    tests, 19–20
Mild hearing loss, 7
Minaural hearing aid, 95
Mixed hearing loss, 11
MMR vaccination, 35
Modem, 122, 127
Moderate hearing loss, 7
Monaural hearing aids, 95
Movies, 137
Muffled sounds, 9
Multiple anomalies, 41
Mumps, 22, 25, 35
Myringoplasty, 57
Myringotomy, 32

National Association for
        Hearing and Speech
        Action, 123
National Board for
        Certification of
        Hearing Instrument
        Sciences (BC-HIS), 77

National Captioning Institute (NCI), 118, 120
  Caption Club, 120
National Center for Law and the Deaf, 130
National Hearing Aid Society, 4, 106
National Information Center on Deafness, 124, 131
National Research Register for Hereditary Hearing Loss, 43, 45
National Society of Genetic Counselors, 43
Nausea, 51, 52
Neck loop, 118
Neomycin, 28, 58
Nerve cells, 46
Nerve deafness, 159. See Sensorineural hearing loss
Newborn intensive-care unit, 41
Noise, 61–70
  and central hearing loss, 11
  danger zone, 63–64, 65
  and head injury, 56
  how to reduce, 69–70
  and job, 63–65
  and sensorineural hearing loss, 10
Noise Control Act (1972), 67
Noise-control laws, 65–67
Noise-reduction circuits, 99
Noise-reduction rating (NRR), 68
Nonorganic hearing loss, 42

Occupational Health and Safety Act (1970), 65, 66–67
Occupational Health and Safety Administration (OSHA), 67
On-the-body hearing aid, 76, 95
Oral contraceptives, 60
Organ of Corti, 23
  and childhood infections, 30, 34
  damage during birth, 27–28
Ossicles (bones in middle ear)
  and conductive hearing loss, 9
  defined, 5–6, 159
  and noise, 62
  testing, 20
  See also Anvil; Hammer; Stirrup
Ossicular chain, 57
Otitis interna, 49–50
Otitis media, 30–32
Otolaryngologist, 14, 16, 46–47
Otologists, 14, 46, 159
Otorhinolaryngologist, 14
Otosclerosis, 9, 53–54
Otoscope, 14–15, 31, 159
Ototoxic drugs, 41, 57–60
  and prenatal hearing loss, 22, 28
Ototoxic jobs, 66
Outer ear, 4–5, 159
Oval window, 159
Oxygen loss, 27–28, 48

Paget's disease, 40
Pain
  in ear, 4
  and hearing aid, 100
Peck, Kathy, 62–63
Pediatrician, 29
Penicillin, 56
Penred's syndrome, 40
Personal FM system (radio-
    frequency aids), 112,
    127, 137
Phone Communicator, 122
Pinna (auricle), 4, **5**, 157, 159
Pitch, 8
Pneumonia, 25
Pot/Trimmer, 89
Pregnant women
  bleeding in, 41
  and CMV exposure, 24–25
  and fetal oxygen, 27–28
  and ototoxic drugs, 28
  and RH factor, 26–27
  and viruses, 25–26
Premature infants, 41, 59
Prenatal hearing loss, 21–29
  and cerebral palsy, 27
  and cytomegalovirus, 23–25
  and group B Streptococcus,
    25–26
  and loss of oxygen, 27–28
  and RH incompatibility, 27
  and rubella, 22–23
  and syphylis, 26
  and toxoplasmosis 23
  and viral infections, 25
Presbycusis
  defined, 1, 45–46, 159

and sensorineural hearing
    loss, 10–11
Pressure
  change, 9
  feeling of, 14, 51
Profound hearing loss, 8
Prolonged labor, 41
Psychogenic hearing loss,
    11–12
  test for, 42
Public meetings, movies and
    concerts, 110, 127,
    136–37
Pure-bone conduction test,
    18
Pure-tone, 159
Pure-tone air-conduction test,
    17–18

Quinidine, 60
Quinine, 59–60

Rabies, 35
Radio-frequency systems
    (personal FM systems),
    137
Reagan, Ronald, 90
Recessive genes, 38–39
Recruitment, 159
Relay services for TTs, 121
Remote control, 89
Resonance, 159
Resources
  for assistive devices, 123–30
  for TT and TDD devices,
    130–34
Rh factor incompatibility,
    26–27, 41

Ringing in ears. *See* Tinnitus
Rock music, 62–63
Rubella (German measles),
        22–23

Salicylate, 59
Scarlet fever (scarlatina), 33
Schools, 16
Scopolamine, 52
Self Help for Hard of Hearing
        People (SHHH), 47,
        48, 131
Semicircular canals, **5**, 6, 160
Senior citizens, 47–48
Sensorineural hearing loss
    causes
        CMV, 23–24
        congenital syphilis, 26
        meningitis, 33
        ototoxic drugs, 28
    defined, 9–11, 160
    and labyrinthitis, 50
    and otosclerosis, 54
    treatment of, 11
Severe hearing loss, 7–8
Sex chromosomes, 39–40
Smoke alarm, 109, 126–29
Social withdrawal, 3
"Sonic Boom" alarm, **109**
Speech
    conservation, 15
    deterioration, 2–3
    discrimination tests, 17, 19
    -reception threshold test,
        18–19
Speech-language pathologist
        (therapist), 160
Speech processor, 103

Speechreading, 143
    and cochlear implants, 105
    training, 15
Stapedectomy, 9, 160
Stapes (stirrup), 5
    otosclerosis and, 53–54
State licensing boards, 77
Steroids, 56
Stirrup, 6, 160
    and noise, 62
Streptomycin, 28, 41, 58
Stroke, 10, 50
Sudden hearing loss, 4
Super-directional
        microphones, 112
Surgery, 20
Syphilis
    and adult hearing loss, 56
    and prenatal hearing loss,
        26, 50
Syphilitic labyrinthitis, 26

Telecaption decoder, 118
    how to buy, 120
    where to get, 126, 127
Telecoil circuitry (T-coil)
    defined, 98–99
    and induction systems,
        110–11
    and infrared systems, 114
    and telephone aids, 114-15
Telecommunications device
        for the deaf (TDD)
    defined, 160
    development of, 121
    how to get information on,
        130–32

where to get, 117, 125–30,
        131–34
    See also Text-telephones
Telecommunications for the
        Deaf, 131
Tele-Consumer Hotline, 117,
        131
Telephone, 114–17
    amplifiers, 116
    and cochlear implants, 105
    and computers, 122–23
    feedback problems, 116
    getting information on, 117
    portable, 115, 116
    telecoil, 114–15
    text-telephone, 121–23
    T-switch compatibility, 115
    where to get aids for,
        124–30
Telephone amplifiers, 124,
        125, 129
Telephone coil, 92
Telephone ring signalers, 109,
        110
    where to get, 124, 126,
        128–29
Television
    closed-caption, 118–20
    devices, 117–18
    infrared listening system,
        113
    and wireless or personal FM
        system, 112
Temporary threshold shift, 64
Text-telephones (TT), 121–23
    how to get information on,
        130–34

Tinnitus (ringing in the ear),
        4, 14, 31, 51, 53
    aids for, 70
    defined, 160–61
    and drugs, 57–58, 59, 60
    and noises, 62
Tobacco, 60
Tobramycin, 28
Touch-Tone phones, 122–23
Toxoplasmosis, 22, 23
Trauma, 52
T-switch, 98, 111
    and telephone, 115
    and TV, 118
TTY, 121, 160. *See also*
        Telecommunications
        device for deaf; Text-
        telephones
Tumors, 11
Tuning fork, 15
TV band radio, 118
Tympanogram, 20
Tympanum. *See* Eardrum

Unilateral functional deafness,
        12
U. S. Congress, 66
United Way, 82
Usher's syndrome, 40

Varicella-zoster virus, 34
Vertigo
    and balance mechanism, 6
    and drugs, 59
    and Menière's disease, 51,
        52–53
    and otosclerosis, 53

Vestibular Menière's disease,
    51
Vestibular testing, 58
Vestibule, **5**, 161
Veterans Administration, 78,
    82
Vibrator, 18
Vibrator alarms, 109–10
Video-cassette recorders
    (VCRs), 118, 127
Viomycin, 58, 59
Viral infections
    and auditory neuritis, 48
    and childhood hearing loss,
        34–35
    and prenatal hearing loss,
        22–26
    and sensorineural hearing
        loss, 10

Viral labyrinthitis, 50
Visual alarms, 108–09, 126
Vowels, 8

Waardenburg's syndrome, 40
Wake-up alarms, 126, 127,
    129
Weitbrecht, Robert, 121
Wireless microphone, 112
Word discrimination
    problems, 10
Word-recognition test, 19

X-linked inheritance pattern,
    39–40

Y chromosome, 39–40
Yellow fever, 35

ⓟ PLUME **DUTTON**

MEDICAL GUIDES

☐ **50 ESSENTIAL THINGS TO DO WHEN THE DOCTOR SAYS IT'S INFERTILITY by B. Blake Levitt.** Whether you have never had a child, or, like many couples, are having difficulty conceiving or carrying a second or third child to term, this essential resource lets you take charge, get started, and determine the best solutions for you. (271193—$10.95)

☐ **SYMPTOMS AND EARLY WARNING SIGNS A *Comprehensive New Guide to More Than 600 Medical Symptoms and What They Mean* by Dr. Michael Apple, Dr. Roy MacGregor, and Dr. Jason Payne-James. Edited by Peter Curtis, M.D., and Carolyn Curtis, R.N.** This indispensable medical reference provides a doctor's approach to diagnosis in a form that makes it easy, accurate, and reliable for the layperson to use. Organized logically from head to toe, according both to major body systems inside and out and to "whole body" symptoms, it gives you fast and easy access to your specific concern. (271134—$15.95)

☐ **THE MOSBY MEDICAL ENCYCLOPEDIA. Revised Edition.** Compiled by a team of leading medical educators working with the nation's foremost medical publisher, this invaluable sourcebook can help you help yourself to better health by providing complete, current information on every significant medical issue. (266726—$19.95)

Prices slightly higher in Canada.

Visa and Mastercard holders can order Plume, Meridian, and Dutton books by calling **1-800-253-6476.**
They are also available at your local bookstore. Allow 4-6 weeks for delivery.
This offer is subject to change without notice.

H1X